Contents

Preface

In the few years since the first edition of this book was published, a great amount of new information – mostly from long-term observational studies and large randomized clinical trials – has become available about the appropriate evaluation and treatment of hypertension in the elderly. This second edition, then, is clearly needed in order to keep practitioners abreast of the developments in this rapidly changing area of clinical medicine.

Introduction

Most people, before they die, will be hypertensive. With life expectancy now being well over 70 in both men and women, the majority of people will develop hypertension before death (Burt et al., 1995; Figure 1).

Most of this hypertension is pure or isolated systolic hypertension (ISH). In the Framingham Study cohort (Kannel, 2000), 60% of those above the age of 65 who had an elevated blood pressure had ISH. This reflects the typical hemodynamic changes occurring with age, which raise

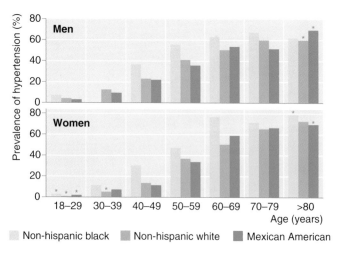

Figure 1 Prevalence of high blood pressure by age and race or ethnicity for men and women in the US population 18 years of age and older. *Estimate based on a sample size that did not meet the minimum requirements of the NHANES III design or relative SEM > 30% date from NHANES III. (From Burt et al., 1995.)

Age (years)	All CV events*		Coronary heart disease		Stroke		Congestive heart failure	
	Men	Women	Men	Women	Men	Women	Men	Women
35–64	18	9	14	6	3	2	3	2
65–94	43	30	27	17	12	11	11	9
Risk ratio	2.4	3.3	1.9	2.8	4.0	5.5	3.7	4.5
65–94/35–64								

*Also includes peripheral vascular disease. CV, cardiovascular.

Table 1 Increment in risk of cardiovascular events in subjects with hypertension comparing age 35–64 year rates in each sex: 36-year follow-up-Framingham study (From Kannel, 1998)

systolic blood pressure and lower diastolic blood pressure as will be noted later.

The presence of hypertension, be it purely systolic or combined systolic and diastolic, poses a major risk to the elderly, both for mortality and even more so for morbidity (Kaplan, 2002). Hypertension remains the major risk factor for strokes, heart failure and coronary disease in the elderly, assuming an even greater role than it does in younger people (Table 1). Whereas diastolic blood pressure is the best predictor of coronary risk in those under 50, systolic pressure and, even more, pulse pressure (the difference between systolic and diastolic pressure) become the major indicators after age 60 (Franklin et al., 2001a).

Fortunately, the treatment of hypertension in the elderly will reduce the morbidities associated with the disease, as will be fully described later. Over the relatively short course (3–7 years) of the randomized controlled trials that have documented the value of antihypertensive therapy, the degree of protection against stroke and, even more so, against heart attack, has been greater in the elderly than in younger patients. The reason is that the inherently greater pretreatment risk status of the elderly provides a greater opportunity for the benefits of blood pressure reduction to be seen than among lower-risk younger patients. Presumably, if younger patients were treated for a much longer period, they would achieve an equal benefit as seen in the elderly over a shorter interval.

Treating the elderly poses a number of special challenges, in both diagnosis and therapy. Fortunately, if these challenges are recognized, most can be met and successful therapy can be provided to most elderly hypertensives.

As a clinician who has worked in the field of hypertension for over 30 years, I appreciate the hurdles that practitioners and patients must overcome to manage the disease appropriately. The remainder of this book will provide the details upon which successful management of hypertension in the elderly can be based.

Mechanisms

Numerous factors, both genetic and acquired, are probably involved in the development of hypertension. Figure 2 is an attempt to integrate some of these factors into a single scheme of pathogenesis. As research increases our understanding, it has become obvious in the majority of hypertensive subjects that no single factor is responsible. One factor rather than another may be of relatively greater importance in some patients, e.g. a reduced nephron number in those who suffered from malnutrition during gestation, resulting in intrauterine growth retardation.

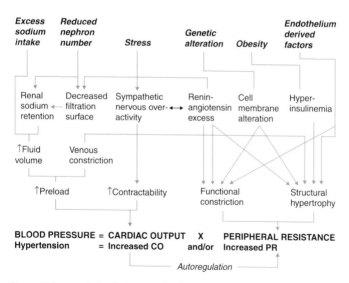

Figure 2 Some of the factors involved in the control of blood pressure that affect the basic equation: blood pressure = cardiac output × peripheral resistance. (From Kaplan, 2002.)

Factors such as obesity, stress or excess sodium intake may all be of particular importance in some patients.

These various factors are involved in the combined systolic and diastolic hypertension that is typical in middle age and which may carry over into old age. About one-third of hypertension in the elderly is of this type, and there is no reason to invoke other pathogenetic mechanisms in those who survive past the age of 65.

Renin in the elderly

As we age, a progressive loss of functioning nephrons occurs: only half of the 800 000 nephrons present at birth typically remain by age 70. As the glomeruli sclerose, the juxtaglomerular (JG) cells lining the afferent arteriole, the source of circulating renin, are also knocked out. In the presence of hypertension an even greater loss of functioning JG cells accompanies the sclerosis of small arterioles that is the hallmark of hypertensive renal damage: benign nephrosclerosis.

The combination of natural aging and hypertensive nephrosclerosis reduces the amount of renin secreted from the kidney. Therefore, the circulating renin level measured as plasma renin activity (PRA) typically decreases in the elderly hypertensive. Black patients with hypertension have even lower PRA levels than non-black patients, either because they are born with fewer nephrons or because they are more susceptible to hypertensive nephrosclerosis.

One possible explanation for the greater extent of renal damage in such patients is an impairment of kidney development during the latter stages of pregnancy. As proposed by Barker and co-workers (Barker, 1995), such intrauterine growth retardation leads to babies who are small for their gestational age. Such small babies grow into adults who have more hypertension, diabetes and coronary disease.

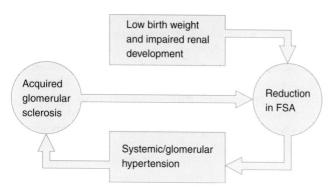

Figure 3 A diagram of the hypothesis that the risks of developing essential hypertension and progressive renal injury in adult life are increased as a result of congenital oligonephropathy, or an inborn deficit of FSA, caused by impaired renal development. Low birthweight, caused by intrauterine growth retardation and/or prematurity, contributes to the oligonephropathy. Systemic and glomerular hypertension in later life results in progressive glomerular sclerosis, further reducing FSA and perpetuating a vicious circle that leads, in the extreme, to end-stage renal failure. (From Brenner and Chertow, 1994.)

Brenner and co-workers (Brenner and Chertow, 1994) believe that reduced renal development is responsible for the subsequent propensity to hypertension (Figure 3). With fewer nephrons, the reduced filtration surface area (FSA) leads to sodium retention and thereby to a rise in systemic blood pressure and subsequently glomerular hypertension. High intraglomerular pressure leads to progressive glomerular sclerosis, setting up a vicious circle: more hypertension causes more glomerular sclerosis, which causes more hypertension.

This scenario almost certainly plays a role in the increased prevalence of subsequent adult hypertension in babies who are small at birth. Whether it is involved in other patients is uncertain, but a tendency for increased renal retention of sodium is likely to be a factor in most hypertension, regardless of how that retention arises.

The low renin levels of older hypertensives might also reflect their tendency to retain sodium, with the subsequent volume expansion raising blood pressure and suppressing the release of renin from the JG cells.

Regardless of how lower renin levels develop, they probably help to explain why the elderly are more responsive to certain drugs (diuretics and calcium antagonists) and less responsive to others (β-blockers and angiotensin-converting enzyme inhibitors (ACEIs) or angiotensin II-receptor blockers (ARBs); (Morgan et al., 2001). Their increased response to diuretics probably reflects their greater initial intravascular volume and their slower and smaller rise in renin when the diuretic contracts intravascular volume and lowers blood pressure, two maneuvers that normally raise renin levels and blunt the continued effect of the diuretic. Because these counter regulatory forces are less active in the elderly, they tend to respond more to the diuretic. A similar mechanism may be at play with calcium antagonists, whose initial effects include a natriuresis.

The smaller response of the elderly and black people to β-blockers, ACEIs, and ARBs probably reflects the fact that all of these agents lower blood pressure at least in part by lowering renin levels or inhibiting renin–angiotensin actions. Therefore, those who start with low renin levels would be expected to respond less to these drugs.

Sodium sensitivity

With fewer functioning nephrons, the elderly hypertensive would be expected to be more sodium sensitive, i.e. have a greater rise in blood pressure when given increased dietary sodium and a greater fall in blood pressure when put on a reduced sodium diet or given a diuretic. Such increased sodium sensitivity has been documented by Weinberger and Fineberg (1991) in a large number of both normotensive and hypertensive patients put through a rapid test of sodium loading and sodium depletion (Figure

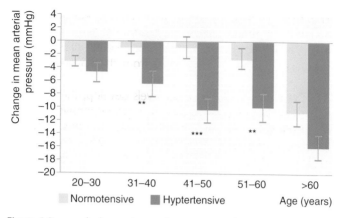

Figure 4 Bar graph shows changes in mean arterial pressure in response to maneuvers used to define salt responsiveness as a function of age in normotensive and hypertensive patients. Standard deviation of the mean given. Significance values between hypertensive and normal subjects. $**P < 0.01$, $***P < 0.001$. (From Weinberger and Fineberg, 1991.)

4). With increasing age, both displayed increasing sodium sensitivity, measured as a greater fall in blood pressure in response to sodium depletion, with the older hypertensives being the most sodium sensitive.

These data are in keeping with the greater response to a sodium-restricted diet in the elderly, as will be described later. They certainly point to a contribution of the usual high sodium intake of most people in modern industrialized societies to the incidence of the hypertension that steadily increases among them. Sodium sensitivity is associated with a higher mortality rate, further emphasizing the need for dietary sodium reduction (Weinberger et al., 2001).

Systolic hypertension

A different scenario probably explains the progressive rise in systolic blood pressure that is the usual form of hypertension

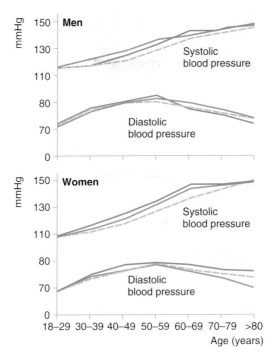

Figure 5 Mean systolic and diastolic blood pressures by age and race or ethnicity for men and women in the US population 18 years of age and older. The red line represents African Americans; the blue line, Mexican Americans; the dashed green line, non-Hispanic Whites. Data from NHANES III survey. (From Burt et al., 1995.)

in the elderly (Figure 5). Systolic blood pressure progressively rises after the age of 50, whereas diastolic blood pressure tends to fall. Part of the fall in the average diastolic blood pressure of the population past the age of 50 can be attributed to the early death from cardiovascular disease of those with significantly high diastolic blood pressure.

The remainder of these diastolic falls with age reflects the basic structural change in the large arteries, the capacitance vessels, which occurs in most people living in industrialized societies, i.e. progressive atherosclerosis (Figure 6). Because

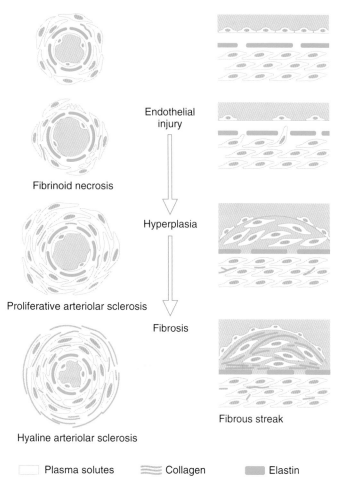

Endothelial
injury

Fibrinoid necrosis

Hyperplasia

Proliferative arteriolar sclerosis

Fibrosis

Hyaline arteriolar sclerosis

Fibrous streak

☐ Plasma solutes   ≋ Collagen   ▬ Elastin

Figure 6 Small vessel arteriosclerosis, or arteriolar sclerosis (left) has many features in common with large vessel atherosclerosis (right). The diagram outlines mechanisms whereby both lesions might originate from a common source (endothelial injury), which leads to the entry of serum factors that stimulate replication of smooth muscle cell in the intima and the formation of an atherosclerotic plaque. In small vessels the result is hypertrophy, hyperplasia and fibrosis of the vascular media. (From Schwartz and Ross, 1985.)

of the reduced caliber of these capacitance vessels, the normal drain-off into the peripheral vasculature during diastole would leave less blood filling those vessels, thereby reducing the pressure within them.

The basic mechanism for the progressive rise in systolic blood pressure with age is the same loss of distensibility and elasticity in the large-capacitance vessels from atherosclerosis. The process was demonstrated over 60 years ago in a simple experiment by Hallock and Benson (1937) (Figure 7). They infused increasing volumes of saline into the tied-off aortas taken from people at autopsy whose ages at death ranged from the early 20s to the late 70s. The pressure within the aortas from the elderly subjects rose much higher with small increases in volume than in younger subjects, reflecting the rigidity of the elderly arteries. A volume little more than normal cardiac output was enough to raise pressure significantly, mimicking the situation during life.

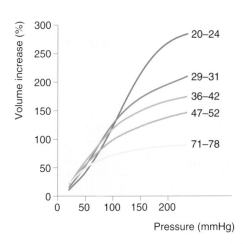

Figure 7 The curves show the relation of the percentage of the increase in volume to the increase in pressure for five different age groups and were constructed from the mean values obtained from a number of aortas excised at autopsy. (From Hallock and Benson, 1937.)

With more sophisticated techniques, the large arteries have been recognized to serve as both conduits and cushions, the first to deliver blood with a minimal fall in pressure to peripheral tissues, the second to smooth out 'the pulsations imposed by the intermittently contracting heart so that blood is directed through these tissues in an almost steady stream' (O'Rourke, 1995). With aging and hypertension, alterations in the cushioning function of the larger arteries occur, changes referred to as 'stiffness' or reduced compliance.

These changes in distensibility and pulse wave velocity that occur with age and which are accentuated by hypertension explain the progressively higher systolic pressures in the elderly. As O'Rourke and co-workers (O'Rourke, 1995) have

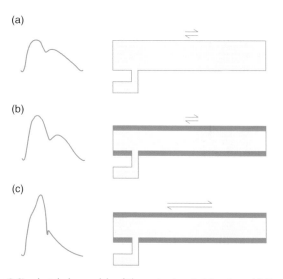

(a)

(b)

(c)

Figure 8 Simple tubular models of the systemic arterial system. (a) Normal distensibility and normal wave velocity; (b) decreased distensibility but normal pulse wave velocity; (c) decreased distensibility with increased pulse wave velocity. At the left are the amplitude and contour of pressure waves that would be generated at the origin of these models by the same ventricular ejection (flow) waves. Decreased distensibility per se increases pressure wave amplitude, whereas increased wave velocity causes the reflected wave to return during ventricular systole. (From O'Rourke, 1995.)

shown, the aortic pulse wave velocity typically doubles by the age of 70 as a manifestation of arterial stiffness from the loss of elastic tissue in the vessel wall. As these pulse waves travel more rapidly and are reflected backwards from the periphery, secondary waves are seen during systole in the elderly (Figure 8). The early return of reflection provides a boost to pressure in late systole, leading to the progressive rise in systolic pressure but a fall in diastolic pressure, widening the pulse pressure. Thereby, typically the blood pressure goes from 120/80 to 170/60 mmHg and often much higher.

Endothelial dysfunction

Over the past 10 years, a virtual explosion of research has transformed our understanding of the vascular endothelium from a passive lining of the blood vessel walls to an active organ, virtually a factory producing various relaxing and constricting factors. The most important of the relaxing factors is nitric oxide, whereas the major constricting factor appears to be endothelin. These various factors are normally in equilibrium, but imbalances may explain both hypo- and hypertension.

The endothelial function in hypertensive but otherwise healthy elderly subjects has generally been found to be no different than that seen in normotensive elderly subjects. However, endothelial dysfunction, as manifested by decreased nitric oxide-mediated vasodilatation, has been noted in a number of conditions that may afflict the elderly. These include hypercholesterolemia, glucose intolerance and insulin resistance, and smoking, and so it would not be surprising that these contribute to hypertension in the elderly.

Other mechanisms

Obviously, the longer we live the greater our exposure to various environmental insults that could damage the heart and vasculature and lead to more hypertension. That fact that only part of the elderly population develops hypertension may reflect differences in genetic endowment or susceptibility to environmental insults. However it arises, hypertension is common and represents the major risk factor for the various cardiovascular complications associated with growing older. The risks imposed by hypertension will be defined next.

Risks

If left untreated, hypertension accelerates atherosclerosis and imposes a further burden on the cardiovascular system (Figure 9). All of these complications occur more frequently in hypertensives, although only accelerated-malignant hypertension and hypertensive encephalopathy are unique to the condition. Those two syndromes were seen in as many as 7% of patients before the advent of effective therapy and were rapidly fatal. Now they are both less common and much more amenable to effective therapy.

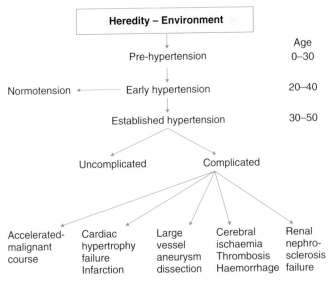

Figure 9 The natural history of untreated essential hypertension. (From Kaplan, 2002.)

Age of onset

In most earlier series of patients observed from the presumed onset of primary or essential hypertension, the age of onset was usually before the age of 50. More recently, however, more representative populations have been witnessed wherein as many as 20% of people who developed diastolic hypertension are over the age of 60. As noted earlier, the overwhelming majority of patients who develop isolated systolic hypertension (ISH) are well over 60, and the majority of hypertensives over the age of 55 have ISH (Franklin et al., 2001b).

In the large population observed by Buck et al. (1987) for 5 years after the onset of combined systolic and diastolic hypertension, the rate of the occurrence of cardiovascular events in these newly diagnosed hypertensives was little higher in those in the 40–49-year age group than in the 60–65 age group (Table 2). However, the odds ratio of events was far greater in the younger hypertensives than in similarly aged normotensives, whereas it was little different between the older hypertensives and older normotensives. As noted by Buck et al. (1987): 'Age overtakes hypertension as a cause of cardiovascular disease'.

Age group (years)	Rate of cardiovascular events per 100 over 5 years*		
	New hypertensives	Normotensive	Odds ratio
40–49	4.6 (239)	0.9 (4677)	5.2
50–59	5.6 (288)	3.2 (3655)	1.8
60–65	6.5 (153)	5.7 (1301)	1.2

*Number of subjects is shown in parentheses.

Table 2 Five-year occurrence of cardiovascular events in newly diagnosed hypertensive subjects and normotensive subjects by age at baseline (data from Buck et al., 1987)

The risks of hypertension in the elderly

None the less, the presence of hypertension poses an additional risk for cardiovascular damage at all ages. Perhaps the clearest portrayal of the progressive increase

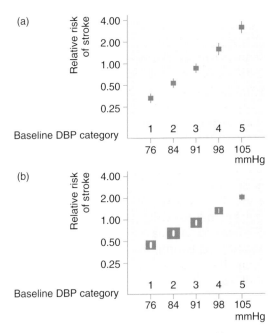

Approximate mean usual DBP (estimated from later remeasurements in the Framingham study)

Figure 10 Relative risk of (a) stroke and (b) CHD, estimated from the combined results of prospective observational studies for five categories of DBP (estimates of the usual DBP in each baseline DBP category are from mean DBP values in the Framingham study recorded 4 years after baseline measurement). The stroke data were obtained from seven prospective observational studies, $n = 843$ events. The CHD data were obtained from nine prospective observational studies, $n = 4856$ events. The solid lines represent disease risk in each category relative to risk in the whole study population (square size is proportional to the number of events in each DBP category). The vertical lines represent 95% confidence intervals for the estimates of relative risk. (From MacMahon et al., 1990.)

in both heart attack and stroke with increasing blood pressure is the analysis of MacMahon et al. (1990) (Figure 10). Their curves are constructed using data from multiple prospective observational studies in which over 450 000 subjects were followed without therapy for variable periods. These relative risk relationships are for diastolic blood pressure but, as we shall see, the degrees of risk are even steeper for systolic blood pressure.

Note in Figure 10 that the increase in the risk for stroke is steeper than for coronary heart disease (CHD) with every increment in blood pressure, but that the number of events, shown as the size of the squares, is much greater for CHD than for stroke. CHD is the leading cause of death in all industrialized societies, but hypertension plays a greater role in the risk for stroke, which is the third leading cause of death overall.

Data from one of the studies that provided most of the numbers shown in Figure 10, the Multiple Risk Factor Intervention Trial (MRFIT) in the US, demonstrate the greater relative risk for CHD with increasing systolic blood pressure than for increasing diastolic blood pressure (Neaton and Wentworth, 1992) (Figure 11). Note the column on the top right representing systolic blood pressure of 160+ and diastolic blood pressure of less than 70 mmHg, the typical pattern of blood pressure in the elderly with isolated systolic hypertension (ISH). This is by far the tallest bar in the figure, documenting the high risk from such elevated systolic levels.

In several placebo-controlled randomized trials involving elderly hypertensives, mortality rates over the 4–5 years of follow-up among those on placebo were similar in those with ISH as in those with combined systolic and diastolic hypertension. Compared to normotensives, those with ISH have more coronary disease and even more strokes, with an approximate 1% increase in all-cause mortality rates with each 1 mm rise in systolic pressure (Staessen et al., 2000).

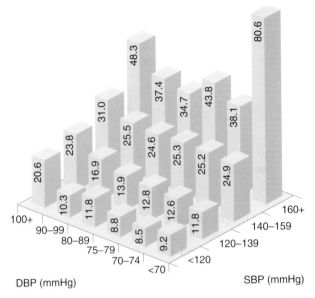

Figure 11 Age-adjusted coronary heart disease death rates per 10 000 person-years by level of SBP and DBP for men screened in the MRFIT. (From Neaton and Wentworth, 1992.)

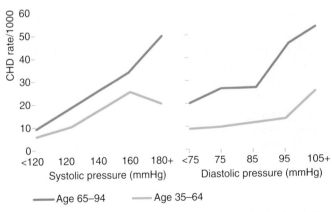

Figure 12 Incidence of coronary heart disease by age levels of systolic blood pressure for a 30-year follow-up in men in the Framingham Study. (From Kannel, 1998.)

Older versus younger

The Framingham data (Kannel, 1998) show the far greater risk for the elderly than for the younger at all levels of both systolic and diastolic pressure (Figure 12). Women have a lower incidence of cardiovascular disease than men do at all ages and with both measures of blood pressure.

The very old

A possible exception to the progressive risks associated with every rise in systolic pressure has been claimed for the very old, i.e. people over the age of 85. Satish et al. (2001) noted better survival in people aged 85 and older with higher initial systolic and diastolic blood pressure than in those with lower readings. This inverse relation may be mainly due to the poor general health that leads to low blood pressure in the elderly.

Hypertension and dementia

Hypertension predisposes the elderly to dementia. This is often vascular in origin, reflecting multiple small infarcts throughout the brain. Fortunately, the incidence of dementia has been found to be reduced in elderly hypertensives given antihypertensive therapy. The most striking effect was reported by Forette et al. (1998) from the SYST-EUR trial of a long-acting dihydropyridine calcium antagonist, nitrendipine. It may be that any effective antihypertensive regimen will protect against vascular dementia as it will against strokes, but that has not yet been shown.

Before considering the ability of antihypertensive therapy to protect the elderly hypertensive, we will consider the measurement of blood pressure and those special features of blood pressure in the elderly, i.e. pseudohypertension and postural hypotension.

Measurement of blood pressure and postural hypotension

Of all the routine procedures performed in clinical practice, measurement of blood pressure (BP) is surely the one that is least accurate but at the same time most important. As stated by O'Brien (1996), 'blood pressure measurement as done in clinical practice today is a very inaccurate procedure, yet one on which we base management decisions with serious far-reaching consequences for the patient'.

Multiple and more accurate blood pressure measurements are needed, primarily because of the marked variability of the blood pressure, as shown in the 24-hour readings taken by an automatic recorder on a single patient taking no medication and performing his usual daily activities (Figure 13). Note the marked difference between the reading taken at 16:30 hrs (160/110 mmHg) and the one taken at 13:30 hrs (120/62 mmHg).

Various extraneous factors could explain this 40/48 mmHg difference between the two readings. They include physical activity, smoking, anxiety, urinary bladder distention, caffeine ingestion, and literally a hundred other factors, many of which cannot be controlled and which are usually not considered. Clearly, if only a few (even accurate) measurements of blood pressure are taken, significant over- and underestimates may be obtained. The only way to overcome the problem of variability is to take multiple readings, following the guidelines as carefully as possible (Beevers et al., 2001) (Table 3, Figure 14).

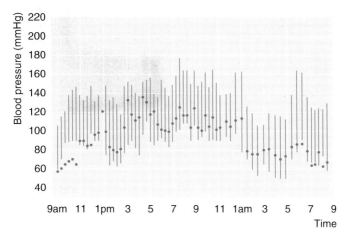

Figure 13 Computer printout of blood pressures obtained by ambulatory blood monitoring over 24 hours, beginning at 09:00 h in a 50-year-old man with hypertension receiving no therapy. The patient slept from midnight until 06:00 h. Heart rate in beats/min. (From Zachariah et al., 1988.)

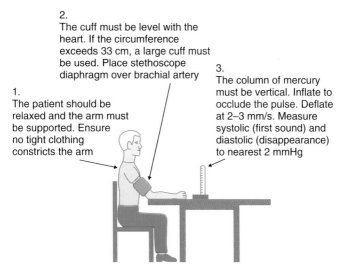

2.
The cuff must be level with the heart. If the circumference exceeds 33 cm, a large cuff must be used. Place stethoscope diaphragm over brachial artery

3.
The column of mercury must be vertical. Inflate to occlude the pulse. Deflate at 2–3 mm/s. Measure systolic (first sound) and diastolic (disappearance) to nearest 2 mmHg

1.
The patient should be relaxed and the arm must be supported. Ensure no tight clothing constricts the arm

Figure 14 Technique of blood pressure measurement recommended by the British Hypertension Society. (From British Hypertension Society, 1985.)

Patient conditions

Posture

- Initially, particularly in patients > 65 years, with diabetes or receiving antihypertensive therapy, check for postural changes by taking readings after 5 minutes supine, then immediately upon and 2 minutes after standing
- For routine follow-up, the patients should sit quietly for 5 minutes with the arm bared and supported at the level of the heart and the back resting against the chair

Circumstances

- No caffeine or smoking within 30 minutes preceding the reading
- No exogenous adrenergic stimulants (e.g. phenylephrine in nasal decongestants)
- A quiet, warm setting

Equipment

Cuff size

- The bladder should encircle at least 80% of the circumference and cover two-thirds of the length of the arm; if it does not, place the bladder over the brachial artery
- A too small bladder may cause falsely high readings

Manometer

- Either a mercury, recently calibrated aneroid or validated electronic device

Stethoscope

- The bell of the stethoscope should be used; to avoid interference, the cuff may be placed with the tubing on the top

Infants

- Use ultrasound (e.g. the Doppler method)

Technique

Number of readings

- On each occasion take at least two readings, separated by as much time as is practical; if readings vary by > 5 mmHg, take additional readings until two are close
- For diagnosis, obtain three sets of readings at least 1 week apart
- Initially, take pressure in both arms; if the pressures differ, use the arm with the higher pressure
- If the arm pressure is elevated, take the pressure in one leg, particularly in patients < 30 years old

Performance

- Inflate the bladder quickly to a pressure 20 mmHg above the systolic pressure, recognized by disappearance of the radial pulse, to avoid an auscultatory gap
- Deflate the bladder 3 mmHg/s
- Record the Korotkoff phase I (appearance) and phase V (disappearance), except in children, for whom use of phase IV (muffling) may be preferable
- If the Korotkoff sounds are weak, have the patient raise the arm and open and close the hand 5–10 times; then inflate the bladder quickly

Recordings

- Note the pressure, patient position, the arm, and cuff size (e.g. 140/90 mmHg, seated, right arm, large, adult cuff)

Table 3 Guidelines for measurement of blood pressure

The white coat effect

Even if all these guidelines are carefully followed, routine clinical measurements by sphygmomanometry will probably display considerable variability. In particular the 'white coat' effect will often result in higher readings in the office than are obtained outside the office. This 'alerting reaction' is partly in response to the presence of the physician and to a lesser degree to a nurse, but more from the anticipation of going to the doctor's office. A good demonstration of the typical differences between office readings and readings taken by the patient at home with an electronic device is shown in Table 4 (Hall et al., 1990). In both the treated and the untreated patients, the first set of clinic readings were higher than the second set taken 2 weeks later, showing the usual fall in blood pressure noted on repeated readings over the first few weeks. Even more impressive is the difference between the clinic readings and the average of 32 self-recorded home readings taken in the 2 weeks between the two office visits, the Home Series in Table 4. The home readings were lower in 80% of the patients – by more than 20/10 mmHg in 40% – so that therapy was deemed unnecessary in 38% of the untreated patients and could be reduced in 16% of the treated ones. The accuracy of the home readings taken with the electronic devices is shown by the identical results with that device and the mercury manometer at the second clinic visit.

White-coat hypertension

Although the blood pressure typically falls over the first few weeks of repeated measurements taken either in the office or at home, in about 20–30% of patients the office readings remain elevated but those taken out of the office are normal. This condition is referred to as 'white-coat hypertension' or 'isolated office hypertension'. The condition was clearly identified by Pickering and co-workers among 292 untreated patients with office readings that were persistently elevated above 140/90 mmHg over an

Patient group	First clinic reading (mercury manometer)		Home series (electronic device)		Second clinic reading (electronic device)		Second clinic reading (mercury manometer)	
	SBP	DBP	SBP	DBP	SBP	DBP	SBP	DBP
Untreated (n = 114)	174	103	148	90	165	95	164	97
Treated (n = 154)	177	104	147	87	163	95	164	95

Data from Hall et al., 1990.

Table 4 Blood pressure recorded at home between clinic visits

average of 6 years (Pickering, 1988). When out-of-office recordings were obtained by 24-hour ambulatory monitoring, the average daytime reading was below 134/90 mmHg in 21% of the patients.

Similar percentages of white-coat hypertension have been noted in various populations all over the world. Interestingly, the prevalence rises with the age of the patient and is particularly high in elderly patients with isolated systolic hypertension. Therefore, it is important to obtain out-of-office readings either by self-recorded home measurements or by ambulatory automatic monitors if at all possible, before diagnosing hypertension in the elderly. Every practitioner should have a few electronic devices to loan to new patients for a few weeks of home recordings. Where feasible, a single 24-hour ambulatory recording will suffice, taking the average of all of the daytime readings, as those taken during sleep are typically lower (see Figure 13) and should not be used in defining the presence of hypertension.

A number of caveats are to be noted concerning white-coat hypertension.

- The prevalence depends on the definition of the upper limit of normal for daytime out-of-office readings. Mancia et al. (1997) recommend 130/85 mmHg, the 95th percentile of a large sample of the population of Monza, Italy.
- A considerable portion of patients considered to be resistant to therapy on the basis of office readings above 140/90 mmHg while on multiple medications have been found to have normal readings when blood pressures are taken out of the office. The appropriate evaluation of such patients is demonstrated in Figure 15. If significant target organ damage is present, more intensive treatment is indicated even if a white-coat component is

making the office pressure higher than it is out of the office. If target organ damage is not present, home blood pressure readings should be obtained and, if they are low, ambulatory monitoring might be considered to document the 'pseudoresistance'. Obviously, if home or ambulatory blood pressures are high, true resistance is confirmed and more intensive therapy should be provided.

- The natural history of white-coat hypertension is under intense scrutiny but has not yet been completely elucidated. Most investigators find a few abnormal features among white-coat hypertensives. However, the longest follow-up of a sizeable group of carefully defined patients with ambulatory readings below 130/80 mmHg shows no increase in cardiovascular events among them compared to a group of patients with normal office and ambulatory readings (Verdecchia et al., 1996; Verdecchia, 2001) (Figure 16). Note that when Verdecchia et al. used a less restrictive higher upper limit of normal to define white-coat hypertension (group C), many of these patients did suffer a cardiovascular event, their probability being close to that seen in the patients with ambulatory hypertension (group D). Clearly, the diagnosis of white-coat hypertension should be restricted to those with truly normal out-of-office readings.

- In keeping with the above caution, if home readings are used, the patient should be instructed to take multiple readings while stressed as well as while relaxed, at home and at work, so as to recognize the true status of the blood pressure. If only relaxed blood pressures are used, many more patients will be thought to have white-coat hypertension than actually do.

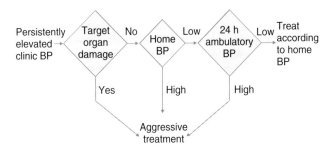

Figure 15 Proposed schema of blood pressure measurement for patients with apparently resistant hypertension. (From Pickering, 1988.)

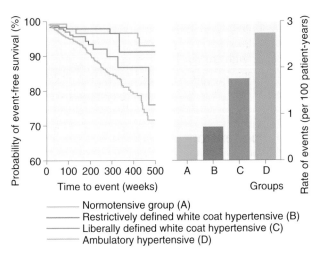

— Normotensive group (A)
— Restrictively defined white coat hypertensive (B)
— Liberally defined white coat hypertensive (C)
— Ambulatory hypertensive (D)

Figure 16 Rate of major cardiovascular morbid events in the normotensive group and in the groups with white-coat and ambulatory hypertension. Event rate did not differ between the normotensive group (A) and the group with more restrictively defined white-coat hypertension (B): daytime ambulatory BP < 130/80 mmHg. Event rate increased in the group with the more liberally defined white-coat hypertension (C). The event rate in group C did not differ from that in the group of patients with ambulatory hypertension (D). (From Verdecchia et al., 1996.)

Currently, the best course is to obtain out-of-office readings to identify white-coat hypertension, as those patients cannot be otherwise recognized. If the patient is truly normotensive out of the office, the diagnosis of hypertension should not be affixed to them, and nor should antihypertensive drug therapy be started. Rather, such patients should be strongly encouraged to modify harmful lifestyle habits (as will be described later) and to monitor their blood pressure carefully as some may progress to persistent hypertension.

Some investigators and practitioners object to this more conservative approach, noting that all of the data on the risks of hypertension have been based on office readings, and often on only a limited number of them. More long-term follow-up is needed but, at present, out-of-office readings have been shown to be more closely predictive of future risk. High office readings are not to be disregarded, but they include some with truly high readings (who are at increased risk) and others with readings that are high because of the white-coat effect (who seem to be at little increased risk).

Pseudohypertension

As noted, the white-coat effect is more common and significant in the elderly than in younger people, and so out-of-office readings should be obtained if possible. In addition to white-coat hypertension, the elderly may have artifactually elevated pressures by usual indirect cuff measurements because of the increased stiffness of the large arteries, which precludes compression and collapse of the brachial artery. Therefore, the manometer shows much higher pressures in the balloon than are present within the artery, giving rise to pseudohypertension. The prevalence varies in various reports, but is probably less than 5%. It should be suspected if high sphygmomanometer readings are noted but few signs of such severe hypertension are present, and particularly if symptoms of hypotension follow only a modest lowering of pressure with antihypertensive therapy. More accurate estimates of true intra-arterial pressure may be obtained by oscillometric measurements.

Postural and postprandial hypotension

Definition and incidence

A fall in systolic pressure of 20 mmHg after 1 minute of quiet standing is usually taken as an abnormal response indicative of postural hypotension. In the generally healthy population of elderly men and women enrolled in the Systolic Hypertension in the Elderly Program, postural hypotension was found in 10.4% at 1 minute after rising from a seated position, and in 12.0% at 3 minutes, with 17.3% having hypotension at one or both intervals. The prevalence would probably have been higher if the patients had been tested after rising from a supine position. The only predisposing factor for postural hypotension found in an unselected elderly population was hypertension. As seen in Figure 17, the higher the basal supine systolic blood pressure, the greater the postural fall.

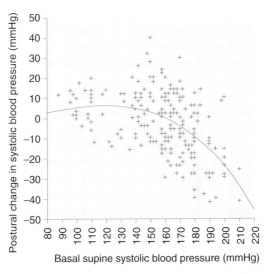

Figure 17 Relationship between basal supine systolic BP and postural change in systolic BP for aggregate data from older subjects. (From Lipsitz et al., 1985.)

Mechanism

Normal aging is associated with various changes that may lead to postural hypotension. The two most common in patients with supine or seated hypertension are venous pooling in the legs and autonomic insufficiency. The reductions in baroreceptor sensitivity that often accompany isolated systolic hypertension are mainly related to aging.

Postprandial hypotension is related to splanchnic pooling of blood after eating. As reported by Grodzicki et al. (1998) among 530 patients aged 60–100 years, ambulatory blood pressure monitoring revealed some decreases in both systolic and diastolic pressure in 70%, the falls being −16/−12 or more in 24%.

Management

Postural and postprandial hypotension must often be treated before the frequently coexisting seated and supine hypertension can be managed (Tonkin, 1995). A summary of the exacerbating factors, pathophysiology and therapy of postural hypotension is shown in Figure 18. A few additional points deserve emphasis.

- A trial of withdrawal of antihypertensive therapy may be worthwhile if simple measures are not effective; however, postural hypotension may improve after effective antihypertensive therapy.
- Simple physical countermeasures often do work, including sleeping with the head tilted up and any isometric exercise before ambulating.
- Drugs that may work include the partial β-agonist pindolol; erythropoietin; the somatostatin analog octreotide, particularly to prevent splanchnic pooling after eating; and the α-agonist midodrine, for those with neurogenic causes.

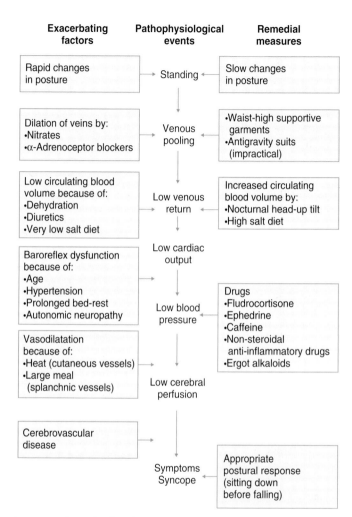

|Exacerbating factors|Pathophysiological events|Remedial measures|

Figure 18 The pathophysiological events during onset of postural hypotension (middle column), the interaction of exacerbating factors (left column) and remedial measures (right column). (From Tonkin, 1995.)

Postprandial hypotension is usually ameliorated by smaller meals, perhaps lower in carbohydrate to minimize the rise in insulin that may induce vasodilation. Caffeine does not prevent postprandial hypotension.

Definition of hypertension

Now that we have reviewed the proper measurement of blood pressure in the elderly, which must obviously include supine and standing readings, attention will be directed to the remainder of the evaluation in those found to be hypertensive, defined as a usual blood pressure above 140/90 mmHg (Table 5). Those with systolic pressure above 140 and diastolic pressure below 90 mmHg are defined as having isolated systolic hypertension (ISH), although in many series ISH is inappropriately reserved only for those with systolic pressure above 160 mmHg.

Category	Systolic (mmHg)	Diastolic (mmHg)
Normal	< 130	< 85
High normal	130–139	85–89
Hypertension		
Stage 1	140–159	90–99
Stage 2	160–179	100–109
Stage 3	> 180	> 110

Data from Joint National Committee 1997.
*These definitions apply to adults who are not taking antihypertensive drugs and who are not actually ill. When systolic and diastolic BP fall into different categories, the higher category should be selected to classify the individual's BP status. Isolated systolic hypertension is defined as SBP > 140 mmHg and DBP <90 mmHg and stage appropriately.
Optimal BP with respect to cardiovascular risk is <120 mmHg systolic and <80 mmHg diastolic.
Based on the average of two or more readings taken at each of two or more visits after an initial screening.

Table 5 Classification of blood pressure for adults aged 18 years and older*

Evaluation

There are three main reasons to evaluate patients with hypertension (Kaplan, 2002).

1. To determine the type of hypertension, looking specifically for reversible causes.
2. To assess the impact of the hypertension on target organs.
3. To estimate the patient's overall risk profile for the development of premature cardiovascular disease.

Such evaluation can be accomplished with relative ease and should be part of the initial examination of every newly discovered hypertensive. The younger the patient and the higher the blood pressure, the more intensive the search for reversible causes should be. Among middle-aged and older patients greater attention should be directed to the overall cardiovascular risk profile, as these populations are more susceptible to immediate catastrophes unless preventive measures are taken.

History

The patient's history should focus on the duration of the blood pressure and any prior treatment, the current use of various drugs that may cause it to rise, and the symptoms of target organ dysfunction (Table 6). Although it is not

Duration of hypertension	Presence of other risk factors
Last known normal blood pressure	Smoking
Course of the blood pressure	Diabetes
Prior treatment of the	Dyslipidemia
hypertension	Physical inactivity
Drugs; types, doses, side effects	**Dietary history**
Intake of agents that may cause	Sodium
hypertension	Alcohol
Oral contraceptives	Saturated fats
Sympathomimetics	**Psychosocial factors**
Adrenal steroids	Family structure
Excessive sodium intake	Work status
Family history	Educational level
Hypertension	**Sexual function**
Premature cardiovascular disease	**Features of sleep apnea**
or death	Early morning headaches
Familial diseases:	Daytime somnolence
Pheochromocytoma, renal	Loud snoring
disease, diabetes, gout	Erratic sleep
Symptoms of secondary causes	**Symptoms of anxiety**
Muscle weakness	(usually associated with
Spells of tachycardia, sweating,	hyperventilation)
tremor	Paresthesias
Thinning of the skin	Dizziness
Flank pain	Palpitations
Symptoms of target organ damage	Atypical chest pain
Headaches	Fatigue
Transient weakness of blindness	
Loss of visual acuity	
Chest pain	
Dyspnea	
Claudication	

Table 6 Important aspects of the history

usually considered part of the initial workup, attention should also be directed toward the patient's psychosocial status, looking for such information as the degree of knowledge about hypertension, the willingness to make necessary changes in lifestyle and to take medication, and the family and job situations. An area of great importance is sexual dysfunction, often neglected until it arises after antihypertensive therapy is given. Erectile dysfunction, often attributed to antihypertensive drugs, may be present in as many as half of untreated, elderly hypertensive men, and is most likely related to their underlying vascular disease.

Physical examination

The physical examination should include a careful search for damage to target organs and for features of various reversible causes (Table 7).

Funduscopic

Only in the optic fundi can small blood vessels be seen with ease, but this requires dilation of the pupil, a procedure that should be more commonly practiced. With the short-acting mydriatic tropicamide 1%, excellent dilation can be achieved in almost 90% of patients within 15 minutes.

Keith, Wagener and Barker, in 1937, originally classified the funduscopic changes but mixed two separate vascular changes: hypertensive neuroretinopathy (hemorrhages, exudates and papilledema) and arteriosclerotic retinopathy

---

Accurate measurement of blood pressure
General appearance: distribution of body fat, skin lesions, muscle
   strength, alertness
Funduscopy
Neck: palpation and ausculation of carotids, thyroid
Heart: size, rhythm, sounds
Lungs: rhonchi, rales
Abdomen: renal masses, bruits over aorta or renal arteries,
   femoral pulses
Extremities: peripheral pulses, edema
Neurological assessment

Table 7 Important aspects of the physical examination

(arteriolar narrowing, arteriovenous nicking and silver wiring). Dodson et al. (1996) proposed a simpler grading system for hypertensive retinopathy: A – (non-malignant), generalized arteriolar narrowing and focal constriction; and B – (malignant), hemorrhages, hard exudates and cotton-wool spots, with or without optic disc swelling (Figures 19 and 20).

Laboratory data

Routine

As described in the Sixth Joint National Committee (1997) report (JNC-6), for most patients a hematocrit, a urine analysis, an automated blood chemistry (glucose, creatinine, electrolytes), a lipid profile (total and high-density lipoprotein cholesterol, triglycerides) and an ECG are all of the routine procedures needed. None of these usually yields abnormal results in the early, uncomplicated phases of essential hypertension, but they should always be obtained for a baseline. Surprisingly, only 17% of general practitioners in several countries routinely obtain even this minimal assessment.

Hypertriglyceridemia and, even more threatening, hyper-cholesterolemia are found more frequently in untreated hypertensives than in normotensives. The prevalence increases with the blood pressure level. The association may, in turn, reflect the quartet of upper body obesity, hyperlipidemia, glucose intolerance and hypertension related to hyperinsulinemia. Lipoprotein (a) levels and certain apolipoprotein (a) isoforms are strong and independent risk factors for coronary disease in hypertensives, so these measurements may be added to the lipid profile.

Hyperuricemia is found in up to half of untreated hypertensives and usually reflects underlying nephrosclerosis. Not only is gout more common in hypertensives, but so

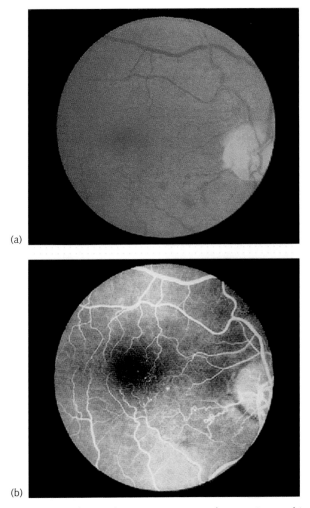

Figure 19 (a) Right eye showing tortuous vessels superotemporal to the optic disc and some microaneurysms close to the fovea, possibly a microvascular occlusion secondary to hypertension. (b) Fluorescein angiogram in the arteriovenous phase of the same patient, showing the tortuous vessels, microaneurysms and dilated capillaries on the nasal side of the foveal arcade. There is also some capillary 'drop out', indicating early ischemia.

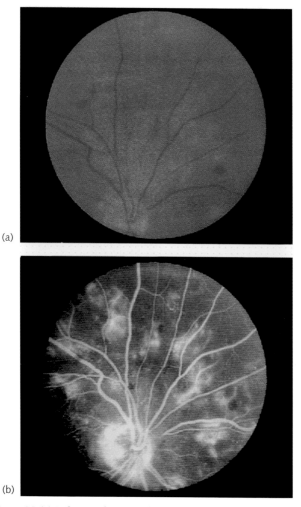

(a)

(b)

Figure 20 (a) Left eye of patient showing numerous cottonwool spots and hemorrhages superonasal to the disc. (b) Fluorescein angiogram in the arteriovenous phase showing masking from the hemorrhages and cottonwool spots. There is leakage from and staining of vessels as they cross poorly perfused areas of the retina. A few microaneurysms can be seen at the top of the picture.

are kidney stones, which are probably a consequence of increased urinary calcium excretion. Incipient renal disease may be heralded by microalbuminuria.

Testing for target organ damage

Left ventricular hypertension hypertrophy (LVH), if significant in degree, can be identified by ECG (Figure 21). Lesser degrees of LVH are identified by echocardiography, but until the recognition of LVH is shown to add independent prognostic information, echocardiography is not recommended as a routine procedure in view of its cost.

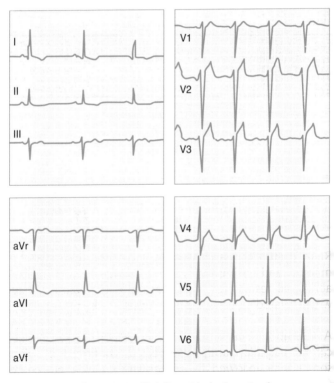

Figure 21 ECG of a patient with left ventricular hypertrophy.

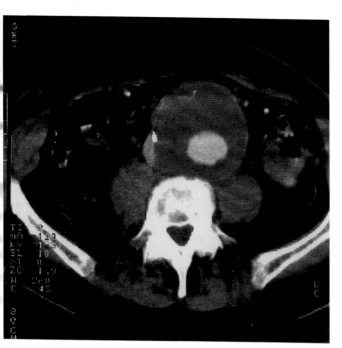

Figure 22 CT scan showing abdominal aortic aneurysm.

In the presence of symptoms of cerebral ischemia the finding of a carotid bruit indicates the need for carotid ultrasonography in the hope of finding a significant and correctable lesion.

Renal dysfunction is usually first recognized by microalbuminuria, and testing for this may become routine. Usually, additional testing for renal damage is reserved for those with elevated serum creatinine levels.

Aortic abdominal aneurysms should be looked for by careful palpation and, if suspected, confirmed by ultrasonography followed by appropriate imaging procedures (Figure 22).

	Diagnostic procedure	
Diagnosis	Initial	Additional
Chronic renal disease	Urinalysis, serum creatinine, renal sonography	Isotopic renogram, renal biopsy
Renovascular disease	Captopril-enhanced isotopic renogram, duplex sonography	CT or MR angiogram Contrast X-ray angiogram
Coarctation	Blood pressure in legs	Aortogram
Primary aldosteronism	Plasma and urinary potassium, plasma renin and aldosterone	Plasma or urinary aldosterone after saline load Adrenal CT and scintiscans Adrenal venous sampling
Cushing's syndrome	Morning plasma cortisol after 1 mg dexamethasone at bedtime	Urinary cortisol after variable doses of dexamethasone Adrenal CT and scintiscans
Pheochromocytoma	Plasma or spot urine for metanephrine	Plasma metanephrine (basal and after 0.3 mg clonidine) Adrenal CT and scintiscans

Table 8 Overall guide to workup for secondary causes of hypertension

Searching for identifiable causes

Evaluation for the major identifiable (or secondary) causes of hypertension is outlined in Table 8. Usually the initial workup for these often reversible causes is limited to patients with features of 'inappropriate' hypertension (Table 9). The one most likely to be found in the elderly is atherosclerotic renovascular disease, particularly when hypertension appears or worsens suddenly and develops on the background of extensive atherosclerotic disease elsewhere. If the initial screening studies are positive or clinical suspicion is strong, the additional studies should be obtained even if initial studies are negative (Vasbinder et al., 2001). The recognition of renal vascular disease is particularly important, as appropriate medical therapy may control hypertension and prevent progressive renal damage (van Jaarsveld et al., 2000).

Sleep apnea is more common in hypertensives and may contribute to resistance to therapy (Lavie and Hoffstein, 2001).

Age on onset: < 20 or > 50 years
Level of blood pressure > 180/110 mmHg
Organ damage
Funduscopy grade II or beyond
Serum creatinine > 1.5 mg/dl
Cardiomegaly or left ventricular hypertrophy as determined by electrocardiography

Presence of features indicative of secondary causes
Unprovoked hypokalemia
Abdominal bruit
Variable pressures, with tachycardia, sweating, tremor
Family history of renal disease

Poor response to generally effective therapy

Table 9 Features of 'inappropriate' hypertension

If identifiable causes seem unlikely on the basis of the history, physical examination and routine laboratory work, the next step is to begin treatment. The evidence that such treatment is beneficial for the elderly with hypertension is examined next.

The benefits of treating hypertension in the elderly

Over the past few years, increasingly strong evidence from large randomized controlled trials (RCTs) has documented the value of treating hypertension in the elderly. Staessen et al. (2000) analyzed the data from eight placebo-controlled randomized trials involving 15 693 elderly patients with ISH (Figure 23). Protection from stroke (a 30% decrease) and coronary disease (a 23% decrease) is quantitatively greater than that shown in multiple RCTs in younger subjects. In particular, the reduction in CHD was almost twice that seen in the younger patients, which is probably a reflection of two factors.

- The elderly start at a much higher risk than the younger and are therefore more likely to achieve benefit over the relatively short duration, i.e. 4–6 years, of these RCTs. If younger patients were treated for 10–20 years they would almost certainly achieve as much benefit.
- Therapy in the more recent RCTs in the elderly was based on low doses of diuretic, which are clearly more cardioprotective than the higher doses of diuretic used in the earlier RCTs in younger patients. As shown by Psaty et al. (1997) (Figure 24), both low doses (up to 25 mg of hydrochlorothiazide or its equivalent) and high doses (50 mg and more) of diuretic provided protection against stroke, as did β-blocker based therapy. For CHD, however, only low-dose diuretic-based therapy has been beneficial.

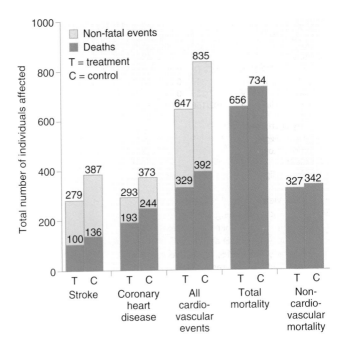

Figure 23 Summarized results in 15 693 older patients with isolated systolic hypertension enrolled in eight trials of antihypertensive drug treatment. Blood pressure at entry averaged 174 mmHg systolic and 83 mmHg diastolic. During follow-up (median 3.8 years) the mean difference in blood pressure between treated and control patients was 10.4 mmHg systolic and 4.1 mmHg diastolic. (From Staessen et al., 2000.)

Results of more recent trials

The 19 RCTs analyzed by Psaty et al. (1997) were published before 1995 and, as noted in Figure 24, all used diuretics and/or β-blockers. Since 1995, an additional 16 RCTs have been completed and analyzed (Blood Pressure Lowering Treatment, 2000). Of these, six compared the newer antihypertensive agents, angiotensin-converting enzyme inhibitors (ACEIs) and calcium antagonists (CAs) against placebo (Table 10).

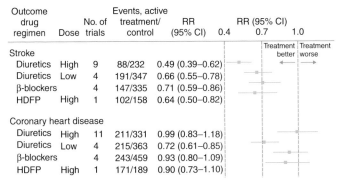

Outcome drug regimen	Dose	No. of trials	Events, active treatment/ control	RR (95% CI)	RR (95% CI)
Stroke					
Diuretics	High	9	88/232	0.49 (0.39–0.62)	
Diuretics	Low	4	191/347	0.66 (0.55–0.78)	
β-blockers		4	147/335	0.71 (0.59–0.86)	
HDFP	High	1	102/158	0.64 (0.50–0.82)	
Coronary heart disease					
Diuretics	High	11	211/331	0.99 (0.83–1.18)	
Diuretics	Low	4	215/363	0.72 (0.61–0.85)	
β-blockers		4	243/459	0.93 (0.80–1.09)	
HDFP	High	1	171/189	0.90 (0.73–1.10)	

Figure 24 Meta-analysis of randomized placebo-controlled clinical trials in hypertension according to first-line treatment strategy. For these comparisons, the number of participants randomized to active therapy and placebo were 7758 and 12 075, respectively, for high-dose diuretic therapy; 4305 and 5116, respectively, for low-dose diuretic therapy; and 6736 and 12 147, respectively, for β-blocker therapy. RR, relative risk; CI, confidence interval. (From Psaty et al., 1997.)

The four RCTs comparing ACEIs against placebo involved patients whose primary problem was coronary disease and not hypertension. The largest by far, the Heart Outcomes Prevention Evaluation (HOPE) trial (2000), included 4355 hypertensive patients, but most were on other antihypertensive drugs and the average blood pressure of the entire 9297 patient population at entry into the trial was only 139/79 mmHg. Despite only a 3/1 mmHg further lowering of BP, significant reductions in all major end-points were seen in those given the ACEI ramipril.

On the other hand, all of the 4695 patients enrolled in the Systolic Hypertension in the Elderly in Europe (Syst-Eur) trial comparing the calcium channel blocker nitrendipine against placebo were hypertensive, and they achieved a 10/5 mmHg fall in BP. Therefore, the somewhat greater benefit against stroke and heart failure found in the CA versus placebo trials than in the ACEI versus placebo trials is not surprising.

	Relative risks (confidence interval)					
	Stroke	CHD	CHF	Major CV events	CV death	Total mortality
ACEI vs placebo (4 trials; 12124 patients)	0.70 (0.57–0.85)	0.80 (0.72–0.8)	0.84 (0.68–1.04)	0.79 (0.73–0.86)	0.74 (0.64–0.85)	0.84 (0.76–0.94)
CA vs placebo (2 trials; 5520 patients)	0.61 (0.44–0.85)	0.79 (0.59–1.06)	0.72 (0.48–1.07)	0.72 (0.59–0.87)	0.72 (0.52–0.87)	0.87 (0.70–1.09)

ACEI, angiotensin-converting enzyme inhibitors; CA, calcium antagonist; CHD, coronary heart disease; CHF, congestive heart failure; CV, cardiovascular.
*Blood Pressure Lowering Treatment Trialists' Collaboration (2000).

Table 10 Prospective overview of randomized trials for hypertension published after 1995*

Additional trials

Two trials not included in the Blood Pressure Lowering Treatment Trialists' Collaboration analysis because of methodological problems have been published, both from China. In the Shanghai Trial of Nifedipine in the Elderly (STONE) (Gong et al., 1996) the patients were entered sequentially and not randomly into the active (nifedipine) or placebo groups, thereby giving rise to possible bias. None the less, the data are quite consistent with the other trials in the elderly, showing significant reductions in stroke and overall mortality with nifedipine (15 deaths in 817 patients) compared to placebo (26 deaths in 815 patients).

Another RCT from China, the Syst-China trial, was designed virtually identically to the Syst-Eur trial and the results are virtually identical: significant reductions in stroke and cardiac events with the long-acting dihydropyridine calcium antagonist nitrendipine compared to placebo in elderly hypertensives (Liu et al., 1998).

β-Blocker based trials

As noted in the Joint National Committee report (JNC-6), but even more definitively shown by Messerli et al. (1998) (Figure 25), the results of the two RCTs in the elderly in which therapy was based on a β-blocker did not show a reduction in coronary events or overall cardio-vascular mortality. There are numerous potential reasons for this inadequacy, as detailed by Messerli et al. As will be seen later, β-blockers are useful drugs in some elderly patients but, as recommended in JNC-6, they should always be combined with a diuretic for the treatment of hypertension, as only such combinations have been shown to be beneficial in the treatment of hypertension in the elderly.

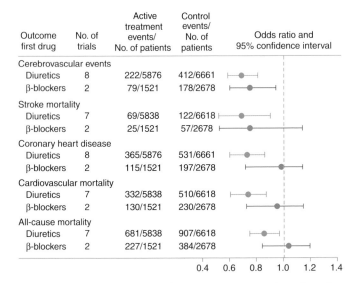

Outcome first drug	No. of trials	Active treatment events/ No. of patients	Control events/ No. of patients	Odds ratio and 95% confidence interval
Cerebrovascular events				
Diuretics	8	222/5876	412/6661	
β-blockers	2	79/1521	178/2678	
Stroke mortality				
Diuretics	7	69/5838	122/6618	
β-blockers	2	25/1521	57/2678	
Coronary heart disease				
Diuretics	8	365/5876	531/6661	
β-blockers	2	115/1521	197/2678	
Cardiovascular mortality				
Diuretics	7	332/5838	510/6618	
β-blockers	2	130/1521	230/2678	
All-cause mortality				
Diuretics	7	681/5838	907/6618	
β-blockers	2	227/1521	384/2678	

Figure 25 Outcome of various end-points in seven or eight trials in the elderly using a diuretic or in two trials using a β-blocker as first drug. (From Messerli et al., 1998.)

When should therapy be started?

In the past, guidelines for the institution of therapy have been based solely on the level of blood pressure, giving rise to major irrationalities and inconsistencies. As noted by Jackson et al. (1993):

'This has led to the situation in which a 60-year-old woman with a DBP of 100 but no other risk factors (her absolute risk of cardiovascular disease is about 10% in 10 years) may meet the criteria for treatment, whereas a 70-year-old man with multiple risk factors but a DBP of 95 mmHg (his absolute risk is about 50% in 10 years) may not.'

On the basis of the results of the multiple clinical trials wherein reductions of blood pressure by about 10/5 mmHg resulted in reductions of overall cardiovascular risk by about one-third, the treatment of these two patients would be expected to reduce the absolute risk in the 60-year-old woman by about 3% in 10 years (30% of 10%), but in the 70-year-old man by about 17% (30% of 50%). As Jackson et al. (1993) note:

> 'In other words, if 100 women aged 60 with DBP of 100 mmHg and no other risk factors were treated for 10 years, about three events would be prevented, whereas if 100 men aged 70 with a DBP of 95 mmHg and multiple other risk factors were treated, about 17 events would be prevented.'

Fortunately, there is now widespread recognition of the need to consider numerous factors beyond just the level of blood pressure in making the decision to treat. JNC-6 provides criteria for three risk groups, based on the level of blood pressure and the presence of major risk factors, such as target organ damage or clinical cardiovascular disease (Table 11). The recommendations are to start therapy in these three groups with either lifestyle modification alone or with drug therapy (Table 12).

Age itself (i.e. over 60 years) is one major risk factor, and most of the elderly with hypertension will have systolics above 160 mmHg so that immediate drug therapy will be indicated for a large proportion. None the less, as we shall see later, lifestyle modifications certainly have an important role in the management of the elderly hypertensive.

The other expert committee guidelines recently published use overall cardiovascular risk as the primary

Major risk factors	Target organ damage/clinical cardiovascular disease
Smoking	Heart disease
Dyslipidemia	Left ventricular hypertrophy
Diabetes mellitus	Angina or prior myocardial infarction
Age > 60 years	Prior coronary revascularization
Sex (men and	Heart failure
postmenopausal women)	Stroke or transient ischemic attack
Family history of	Nephropathy
cardiovascular disease:	Peripheral arterial disease
Women > 65 years or	Retinopathy
men < 55 years	

Table 11 Components of cardiovascular risk stratification in patients with hypertension

Characteristics	Risk group A	Risk group B	Risk group C
Major risk factors	–	+	–/+
Target organ damage or clinical cardiovascular disease	–	–	+
Blood pressure mmHg (stages)			
130–139/85–89 (high-normal)	Lifestyle modification	Lifestyle modification	Drug therapy
140–159/90–99 (stage 1)	Lifestyle modification (up to 12 months)	Lifestyle modification up to (6 months)	Drug therapy
< 160/> 100 (stages 2 and 3)	Drug therapy	Drug therapy	Drug therapy

Table 12 Risk stratification and treatment

criterion for the decision to start antihypertensive therapy (Ramsay et al., 1999; Guidelines Subcommittee, 1999).

Is there an age limit for therapy?

None of the RCTs in the elderly included enough patients over the age of 80 to determine the value of antihypertensive therapy in such patients, the most rapidly growing part of our population. However, almost 1600 patients over age 80 were included in the various trials in the elderly, and they achieved similar protection against stroke and CHD as the less elderly, but not a reduction in mortality (Gueyffier et al., 1999). Until trials now in progress provide definite evidence, the best course is to treat – ever so gently – very old patients with systolic blood pressure above 160 mmHg or diastolic above 90 mmHg if they seem likely to have more than 1 year of life survival. Those who are severely debilitated with end-stage cancer or dementia are best left untreated. However, a 100-year-old who can be protected from stroke or dementia and thereby allowed to maintain an enjoyable life should not be denied such benefit.

Furthermore, there seems no reason to stop successful and well-tolerated therapy, regardless of the attained age. As will be noted later, almost all who are hypertensive before treatment will become hypertensive again if treatment is stopped. If blood pressure becomes lower than 140/85 mmHg, treatment logically should be reduced so as not to keep blood pressure below the level needed for adequate tissue perfusion.

The goal of therapy

Perhaps the issue of how far to reduce the blood pressure should come after the details on therapy, but establishing the goal of therapy is an essential aspect of treatment and should be established 'up front'.

There are three possible relationships between the levels of blood pressure achieved by therapy and the risk of

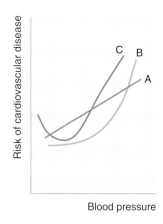

Figure 26 Three models of hypothetical relationships between levels of blood pressure and risk of cardiovascular disease. (From Epstein, 1980.)

cardiovascular disease (Figure 26). Line A implies the lower the blood pressure, the less the risk, in keeping with the straight-line relationship between untreated levels of blood pressure and risk shown in Figure 10. However, the results of the multiple RCTs described earlier have suggested that the consequences of therapy are more accurately portrayed as either line B, wherein little if any additional benefit is derived from increasingly greater reduction in blood pressure, or line C, wherein additional risks appear as the pressure is reduced below some initial level. As is obvious, line C delineates a 'J-curve', the term used for the third scenario.

From the time in 1979 when the English practitioner I.M.G. Stewart reported a fivefold increase in heart attacks among patients whose diastolic blood pressure (fourth Korotkoff phase) was reduced below 90 mmHg, considerable arguments have either defended or denied the presence of a J-curve. The reason for so much discussion is the implication that therapy beyond a certain level could have serious adverse consequences.

The massive Hypertension Optimal Treatment (HOT) trial (Hansson et al., 1998) was designed primarily to answer the issue in a prospective manner, as most of the data for and against the J-curve were retrospective analyses of small numbers of patients. The HOT trial involved almost 19 000 hypertensives aged 50–80 years (mean 61.5 years) with diastolic blood pressure between 100 and 115 mmHg while on no therapy. They were randomly divided into three groups to receive drug therapy adequate to lower their diastolic blood pressure to either 90, 85 or 80 mmHg. Therapy began with the long-acting dihydropyridine calcium antagonist felodipine, and other drugs (ACE inhibitor, β-blocker, diuretic) could be added to achieve the target blood pressure.

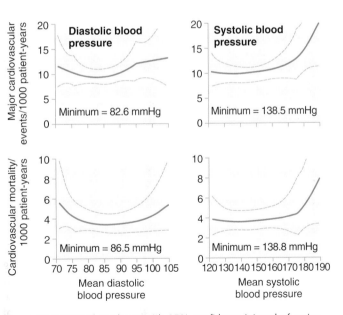

Figure 27 Estimated incidence with 95% confidence interval of major cardiovascular events (top) and cardiovascular mortality (bottom) in relation to achieved mean diastolic and systolic blood pressure in the HOT trial. (From Hansson et al., 1998.)

Unfortunately, at the end of the average 3.8-year follow-up, the separation between the three groups was less than half of the 10 mmHg desired. Therefore, the existence of a J-curve could be neither denied nor documented because of the small degree of blood pressure differences. None the less, when all of the data were analyzed, the relation between achieved blood pressure and cardiovascular risk did show that the 'best' blood pressure with the minimum number of major adverse events was 138.5/82.6 mmHg (Figure 27). No additional benefit was seen at lower pressures. The authors of the HOT trial paper provide arguments against the J-curve. However, a closer look at Figure 27 shows a rise – slight but definite – in cardio-vascular event and mortality at diastolic pressures below 85 mmHg.

Evidence for a J-curve for diastolic pressure

The patients enrolled in the HOT trial had combined systolic and diastolic hypertension. As previously noted, the largest part of the elderly hypertensive population has isolated systolic hypertension (ISH), starting with diastolic BP below 90 mmHg. As also previously noted, the pressure fall in diastolic BP typically occurring over age 55 is, in itself, a risk factor. There is some evidence that further inadvertent reductions in diastolic BP by drug therapy of ISH may increase the risk of stroke.

First, in the SHEP trial, wherein starting BPs averaged 170/77 mmHg, diuretic-based therapy achieved an average 25/7 mmHg fall in BP and, thereby, a significant reduction in stroke and other cardiovascular events (SHEP Cooperative Research Group, 1991). However, subsequent analysis found an increase in stroke events in those whose diastolic BP was reduced more than 5 mmHg and to below 65 mmHg, compared to those with a lesser fall in diastolic levels (Somes et al., 1999).

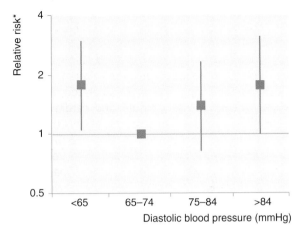

Figure 28 Association between diastolic blood pressure and risk of first-ever stroke in 2351 elderly hypertensives who were using antihypertensive drugs. Reference category is the second lowest category of diastolic blood pressure. Values are plotted on a logarithmic scale. *Adjusted for age, gender, smoking habit, diabetes mellitus, ankle-to-arm index, minor vascular events (intermittent claudication, angina pectoris, history of coronary revascularization procedure), myocardial infarction, atrial fibrillation, and typical and atypical transient ischemic attack. (Modified from Vokó, et al., 1999.)

Second, in a large group of hypertensives observed either with or without antihypertensive drug therapy, those given drugs whose diastolic BP fell below 65 mmHg had an increased number of strokes (Vokó et al., 1999) (Figure 28).

Varying goals

Based on these data, the goal for the elderly with ISH should be a systolic of 140 mmHg, as long as the diastolic does not fall to below 65 mmHg (Staessen et al., 2001). For the elderly with combined systolic and diastolic hypertension, the goal should be 140/85 mmHg. For those with diabetes, renal insufficiency and other high-risk factors, further reductions should be attempted, probably to below 130/80 mmHg.

We will now turn to the therapies that will be needed to reach these goals, starting with lifestyle modifications and then drug therapy.

Therapy: lifestyle modifications

A number of lifestyle changes are known to lower blood pressure in a significant proportion of the hypertensive population (Joint National Committee, 1997) (Table 13). Not all of these have been studied in elderly patients, but their benefits almost certainly apply to them equally as much or even more. For instance, elderly people respond better to a lower sodium intake, i.e. they are more sodium sensitive, as noted earlier (see Figure 4).

Avoidance of tobacco

Nicotine has an acute and often dramatic pressor effect that does not lessen with continued exposure. Tolerance to

Stop smoking
Lose weight if overweight
Limit alcohol intake to ≤ 1 ounce/day of ethanol
  (24 ounces of beer, 8 ounces of wine, or 2 ounces of
  100-proof whiskey)
Reduce sodium intake to 110 mmol/day (2.4 g sodium or 6 g
  sodium chloride)
Maintain adequate dietary potassium, calcium, and magnesium
  intake
Reduce dietary saturated fat and cholesterol intake for overall
  cardiovascular health
Exercise (aerobic) regularly

Table 13 Lifestyle modifications for hypertension

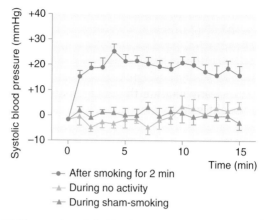

Figure 29 Changes in systolic blood pressure over 15 minutes after smoking the first cigarette of the day in 10 normotensive smokers. (From Groppelli et al., 1992.)

many of the other noxious effects of nicotine develops, but the rise in blood pressure occurs with every exposure (Groppelli et al., 1992) (Figure 29). The pressor effect noted in addicted smokers from the cigarette smoked for 2 minutes is shown to persist for 15 minutes in Figure 29, but is gone by 30 minutes. Therefore, the effect may not be recognized, as smoking is not allowed in clinics or offices where blood pressure is measured. The time from the last puff in the parking lot to the measurement of blood pressure may be far greater than the duration of the last puff's pressor effect. Therefore, if possible, smokers should take their blood pressure while smoking. That reading should be the basis for deciding on therapy and the goal of therapy. Regardless of age or duration of smoking, every effort should be made to get the patient to stop smoking.

Weight loss

Weight gain is the most common direct environmental cause of hypertension. Even relatively small amounts of weight gain increase the incidence of hypertension, as shown in the report by Huang et al. (1998) of a 20-year follow-up of 82 000 US nurses. Those who gained as little as 5 kg (11 lb) from their weight at age 18 had twice as much hypertension as those whose weight did not change; with a 10 kg (22 lb) weight gain the incidence tripled. These data clearly indicate the major contribution of even modest weight gain to the risk for hypertension.

Furthermore, those who lost weight had less hypertension, in keeping with a large body of data showing falls in blood pressure with weight loss (Figure 30). Difficult as it may

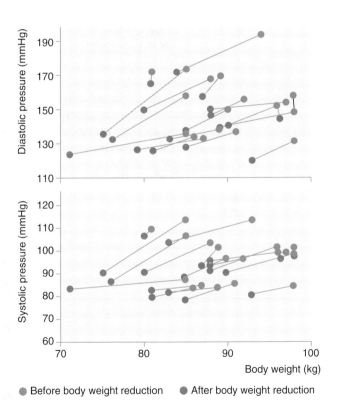

● Before body weight reduction   ● After body weight reduction

Figure 30 Systolic and diastolic blood pressure before and after body weight reduction. (From Staessen et al., 1989.)

be, particularly for the elderly, weight loss must be constantly urged on all overweight hypertensives, and they should be given appropriate dietary advice. The short-term use of diet pills may be of some help, but caution is needed as most can raise blood pressure.

Sodium restriction

Despite a claim based on flawed data by Alderman et al. (1998) that coronary risk was increased among those who ingested a low-sodium diet, the evidence is overwhelming that modest sodium restriction is both safe and effective in lowering blood pressure. Numerous meta-analyses of

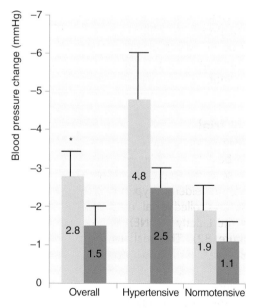

Figure 31 Mean net changes in systolic (pink bars) and diastolic (blue bars) blood pressure, with 95% confidence intervals, pooled for all sodium-reduction trials and for various subsets. *Mean change compared with control, with upper 95% confidence interval. (Modified from Cutler et al., 1997.)

controlled trials have shown a small but significant and almost uniform lowering of blood pressure by a 40–60 mmol/day reduction in sodium intake, approximating the usual recommendation of a 100–110 mmol/day intake (Cutler et al., 1997) (Figure 31).

The elderly are more sodium sensitive and therefore more likely to respond favorably to sodium reduction. However, two factors may make it more difficult for them to reduce sodium: first, taste sensation may diminish with age, and so more salt may be added to achieve the desired degree of saltiness; second, the elderly may be more dependent on processed and packaged foods, which usually have large amounts of sodium added.

The effort to reduce dietary sodium moderately is worthwhile and success can be achieved with counseling, the avoidance of processed foods with more than 300 mg of sodium per portion as indicated on the label (a major boon to sodium avoidance), and occasional checks of urinary sodium excretion.

The TONE trial

Perhaps the best documentation of the benefits and safety of modest sodium restriction, alone or combined with weight loss, in elderly hypertensives comes from the randomized controlled Trial of Nonpharmacologic Interventions in the Elderly (TONE) reported by Whelton et al. (1998) (Figure 32). The trial involved men and women aged 60–80 years with hypertension that was being well controlled on one or two medications. The patients agreed to discontinue their drugs and were then randomly allocated to four groups: (1) no changes, i.e. usual care; (2) modest dietary sodium restriction; (3) weight loss by caloric restriction and increased physical activity; and (4) both sodium restriction and weight loss. Over a 30-month follow-up the patients achieved only modest reductions in

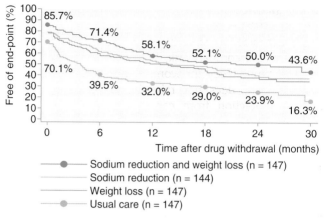

Figure 32 Percentage of the participants assigned to both sodium restriction and weight loss, to sodium restriction alone, to weight loss alone, and to usual care (no intervention) who remained free of cardiovascular events and recurrence of hypertension during the 30-month follow-up of the TONE study. (From Whelton et al., 1998.)

sodium intake (an average of 40 mmol/day) and weight loss (an average of 4.7 kg or 10.3 lb). Despite these modest changes, the number whose hypertension reappeared (the primary end-point) and who developed cardiovascular complications was far greater among the usual care group than among those who reduced either sodium intake or body weight. Those who did both were protected even more.

Subsequent analysis of the TONE data showed that compared to those on usual care, those assigned to sodium reduction achieved a 4.3/2.0 mmHg greater fall in BP accompanied by a 32% reduction in cardiovascular events (Appel et al., 2001).

The TONE data are particularly meaningful because the trial involved 681 elderly hypertensives, it went on for 30 months and it documented the benefits of only modest lifestyle changes that should be achievable in the 'real world'.

Limit alcohol intake

Too much alcohol raises blood pressure (Figure 33); too little increases coronary risk. The appropriate amount, i.e. one-half portion/day for women and up to two portions/day for men, does not raise blood pressure but does provide protection from coronary mortality. (A portion contains 10–12 ml of ethanol = 1.5 ounces of 100 proof spirits, 4 ounces of wine, 12 ounces of beer).

Too much alcohol is probably the most common cause of easily reversible hypertension, the estimate being 8% of hypertensive men in the US (Kaplan, 2002). Those who drink more than two portions on average per day must be strongly advised to cut back.

Small amounts of daily alcohol consumption protect against coronary mortality, as shown in numerous surveys, including that of Thun et al. (1997), who followed 490 000 men

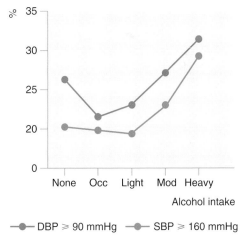

Figure 33 Age-adjusted prevalence rates (%) of measured systolic and diastolic hypertension by levels of alcohol intake in drinks. Occ, occasional; light, one to two daily; Mod, moderate, three to six daily; Heavy, more than six daily. (From Shaper et al., 1988.)

and women for 9 years after ascertainment of their alcohol use. All-cause and cardiovascular mortality was reduced by 30–40% in those who had at least one drink daily, compared to those who did not drink. As expected, mortality from alcohol-related diseases increased with excessive consumption.

The lower recommendation for women should circumvent any threat of stimulation of breast cancer by alcohol.

Maintain adequate dietary potassium, calcium and magnesium

Intake of these three minerals should be well maintained in the elderly, preferably by a diet containing adequate amounts of fresh fruits, vegetables and dairy products; if not, by mineral and vitamin supplements.

An increased intake of 40–80 mmol/day of potassium, preferably in fresh fruits and vegetables, will lower blood pressure almost as much as will moderate sodium restriction, and reduces the risk for stroke (He and MacGregor 2001). On the other hand, as reviewed by Sacks et al (1998), increased intake of calcium or magnesium will not affect blood pressure even in those with low habitual intakes.

More fresh fruits and vegetables reduce BP (Sacks et al. 2001) and the risk for ischemic stroke (Joshipura et al. 1999). These benefits may reflect many effects of such a diet: more fiber, potassium, magnesium and calcium, and less sodium.

Exercise regularly

Of the entire 'lifestyle prescription', regular physical activity may be the most difficult to accomplish in this world of 'couch potatoes' but the one that will provide the most benefit. As shown by Hakim et al. (1998) in their study of older physically capable men, regular walking reduces overall mortality. The longer the walk, the lower the mortality.

Such low-intensity activity will also lower blood pressure, probably contributing to the overall reduction in mortality. Higher-intensity activity may be even better, both to aid in weight loss and to lower blood pressure. Pure isometric exercise (weightlifting) only raises blood pressure acutely; during aerobic or isotonic activity (running, swimming) systolic blood pressure increases and diastolic goes down. Afterwards both systolic and diastolic levels tend to remain lower.

Those elderly hypertensives who cannot walk, run or swim should be encouraged to use whatever exercise devices they can that are available at health clubs and retirement centers.

Reduce dietary saturated fat and cholesterol

There is very likely some benefit on the blood pressure when diet or statin drug therapy lowers serum LDL cholesterol. The effect is mediated by improvements in endothelial function, with increased synthesis of vasodilatory nitric oxide. In most trials of lipid-lowering agents a slight but significant fall in blood pressure has been observed (Goode et al., 1995).

Other modalities

Increased amounts of fiber, omega-3 fatty acids, garlic or oral antioxidants, as well as various relaxation techniques, have been claimed to lower blood pressure, but most of the trials are small, short and poorly controlled (Kaplan,

2002). None of these should have adverse effects, but do not expect them to lower blood pressure.

Two additional drugs are widely used among elderly hypertensives: aspirin and estrogens as replacement therapy (ERT). Aspirin, 75 mg daily, was shown in the HOT trial to reduce coronary events but to increase non-fatal bleeding episodes. ERT, unlike oral contraceptives, does not raise blood pressure and can be given to hypertensive women without concern about their blood pressure.

After these lifestyle changes have been attempted, the blood pressure may remain above the goal, making drug therapy compulsory.

Drug therapy

Treatment of hypertension in the elderly differs in a number of both obvious and subtle ways from the treatment of younger patients. Partly as a reflection of the different pathophysiology described earlier, but mainly because of the multiple 'natural' changes occurring with age, the elderly need to be treated cautiously, following the admonition: 'start low and go slow'.

Because the elderly may have sluggish baroreceptor and sympathetic nervous responsiveness as well as impaired cerebral autoregulation, therapy should be gentle and gradual, avoiding drugs that are likely to cause postural hypotension or to exacerbate other common problems often seen among the elderly (Table 14).

Factors	Potential complications
Diminished baroreceptor activity	Orthostatic hypotension
Impaired cerebral autoregulation	Cerebral ischemia with small falls in systemic pressure
Decreased intravascular volume	Orthostatic hypotension, volume depletion, hyponatremia
Sensitivity to hypokalemia	Arrhythmia, muscular weakness
Decreased renal and hepatic function	Drug accumulation
Polypharmacy	Drug interactions, in particular with non-steroidal anti-inflammatory drugs
CNS changes	Depression, confusion

Table 14 Factors that *might* contribute to increased risk of pharmacological treatment of hypertension in the elderly

These cautions should not, however, interfere with the well-documented need to treat the overwhelming majority of elderly hypertensives. The benefits they have been shown to receive from antihypertensive drug therapy, detailed earlier, are quantitatively greater than those provided to younger patients. No longer should age alone interfere with the provision of appropriate therapy.

General guidelines

The treatment algorithm shown in Figure 34 is well suited to the elderly hypertensive, with the caveat that most wi

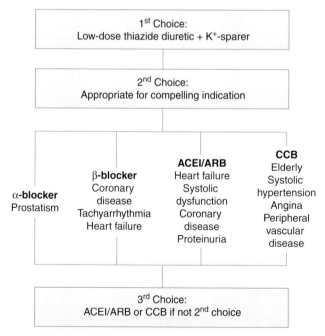

Figure 34 Treatment algorithm based upon the use of a low dose of diuretic as the first choice and, if BP control is not achieved, the addition of a second drug determined by the presence of compelling indications.

have one or more of the compelling and specific indications listed in both the JNC-6 report (1997) and the WHO-ISH guidelines (Guidelines Subcommittee, 1999). As the majority of the elderly will have isolated systolic hypertension, attention will be directed to the compelling indications for diuretics as the preferred initial therapy, and the use of long-acting dihydropyridine (DHP) calcium antagonists as an appropriate second drug or, rarely, an alternative. On the other hand, the striking reduction in recurrent strokes seen in the PROGRESS trial (2001) with a diuretic (indapamide) and an ACEI (perindopril) supports their use in this highly vulnerable group.

Diuretics for initial therapy

As shown earlier, a low-dose diuretic was the first drug used in most of the major randomized controlled trials in the elderly. A large amount of data from the Systolic Hypertension in the Elderly (SHEP) trial has confirmed the efficacy and safety of the step 1 drug chlorthalidone, started at 12.5 mg/day and increased if needed to 25 mg/day. As reported by Savage et al. (1998), this low-dose diuretic regimen was well tolerated and effective in reducing blood pressure by 13/4 mmHg below that noted in the placebo-treated half. Biochemical changes were relatively minimal over the 3 years of active therapy (Table 15). New-onset

Active treatment compared to placebo		
Fasting glucose	+0.20 mmol/l	(+3.6 mg/dl)
Total cholesterol	+0.09 mmol/l	(+3.5 mg/dl)
HDL-cholesterol	–0.02 mmol/l	(–0.77 mg/dl)
Triglycerides	+0.9 mmol/l	(+17 mg/dl)
Creatinine	+2.8 µmol/l	+(0.03 mg/dl)
Uric acid	+35 µmol/l	(+0.6 mg/dl)
Potassium	–0.3 mmol/l	

Table 15 Changes in blood chemistries in the SHEP trial (data from Savage et al., 1998)

diabetes occurred in 8.6% of the diuretic-treated subjects compared to 7.5% of the placebo group.

In a substudy of the SHEP trial reported by Ofili et al. (1998), the low-dose diuretic regimen induced a significant 13% reduction in left ventricular mass, as assessed by echocardiography, whereas a 6% increase in left ventricular mass was noted in the placebo group over the 3-year follow-up.

These data, along with those from the other RCTs described earlier, strongly support the preference given to low-dose diuretics for the elderly. Emphasis should be given to the low doses, equivalent to 12.5 mg of hydrochlorthiazide used as initial therapy, an amount that in itself provided adequate antihypertensive efficacy in about half of the participants.

Long-acting dihydropyridine calcium antagonists

As described earlier, four RCTs have been completed comparing one of these agents against placebo in elderly patients with isolated systolic hypertension (ISH). The two RCTs from China have seemingly had much less impact than the Syst-Eur trial reported by Staessen and co-workers. All three showed excellent protection from both stroke and coronary disease with either long-acting nitrendipine or nifedipine.

The cardioprotection provided by these long-acting DHP calcium antagonists should allay any concerns about the danger noted with very large doses of short-acting nifedipine in the highly vulnerable post myocardial infarction period (Brown et al., 2000). Long-acting antagonists do not lower blood pressure abruptly, thereby avoiding the activation of sympathetic activity that is seen with short-acting agents (Grossman and Messerli, 1997).

Another concern about short-acting calcium antagonists – their promotion of cancer – as reported in retrospective uncontrolled observations has also been clearly documented not to apply to the long-acting agents. In the Syst-Eur trial (Staessen et al., 1997), 15% fewer cancers were diagnosed in those on nitrendipine than in those on placebo. Numerous large surveys have documented the absence of any relationship between calcium antagonists and cancer (Kizer and Kimmel, 2001).

Because nitrendipine is not marketed in the US (or the UK), the JNC-6 report considered the other long-acting DHP calcium antagonists that are available to be appropriate alternatives. These include amlodipine, felodipine, nicardipine, nifedipine XL and nisoldipine.

Comparative trials

Eight trials have been published comparing regimens based on diuretic either with or without β-blockers, ACEIs or CAs (Table 16). One conclusion seems obvious: neither ACEIs nor calcium antagonists are better overall than are diuretics, with or without β-blockers. Certainly, calcium antagonist-based therapy protected better against stroke and less well against CHD and CHF, but the two forms of therapy were identical in their effects on overall morbidity and mortality rates. Furthermore, a good deal of admixture occurred in these trials. In one (Estacio et al., 1998), only 45% of patients assigned to one form of therapy remained on that drug to the end of the trial. In most, approximately 75% did so, but many also took drugs additional to the monotherapy originally started.

Table 16 shows data from the two trials that directly compared an ACEI with a calcium antagonist (Estacio et al., 1998; Hansson et al., 1999). The ABCD trial (Estacio et al., 1998) had 470 patients and the Swedish Trial in Old Patients with Hypertension-2 (STOP-2) (Hansson et al., 1999) had 4401 taking one or the other of these two classes of drugs, so obviously most of the results are

	Stroke	CHD	CHF	Major CV events	CV death	Total mortality
			Relative risks (confidence interval)			
ACEI vs D/βB (3 trials; 16 161 patients)	1.05 (0.92–1.19)	1.00 (0.88–1.14)	0.92 (0.77–1.09)	1.00 (0.93–1.08)	1.00 (0.87–1.15)	1.03 (0.75–0.94)
CA vs D/βB (5 trials; 23 454 patients)	0.87 (0.77–0.98)	1.12 (1.0–1.26)	1.12 (0.95–1.33)	1.02 (0.95–1.10)	1.05 (0.92–1.2)	1.01 (0.92–1.11)
ACEI vs CA (2 trials; 4871 patients)	1.02 (0.85–1.21)	0.81 (0.68–1.0)	0.82 (0.67–1.0)	0.92 (0.83–1.01)	1.04 (0.87–1.24)	1.03 (0.91–1.18)

ACEI, angiotensin-converting enzyme inhibitors; CA, calcium antagonist; CHD, coronary heart disease; CHF, congestive heart failure; CV, cardiovascular; D/βB, diuretic and/or β-blocker.
*Blood Pressure Lowering Treatment Trialists' Collaboration (2000).

Table 16 Prospective overview of randomized trials for hypertension published after 1995*

derived from STOP-2. Although some would make a great deal of the apparent lesser protection against CHD and CHF afforded by the calcium antagonist than the ACEI, the words of the principal investigators of STOP-2 should be heeded: 'Our results should be interpreted with some caution, since 48 statistical comparisons were done. Calcium antagonists were not, however, less effective in any other way in the prevention of cardiovascular events than conventional drugs or ACE inhibitors, which accords with current opinion about safety of calcium antagonists when used appropriately' (Hansson et al., 1999).

The results of the trials completed since 1995 are by no means definitive. As He and Whelton (2000) noted: 'Most of the uncertainties related to selection of initial antihypertensive drug therapy will be resolved by trials in progress and by the pooling of the findings from these trials'. Fortunately, many trials are in progress, so that more definitive data to guide our choices of therapy will soon be available.

Of course, the playing field keeps growing. By the time we know whether ARBs are as good as ACEIs, vasopeptidase inhibitors will probably be available, so the process of finding out what is best will probably never end.

In one sense the process is irrelevant. As the need to achieve lower goals of therapy has become obvious, the need to use more than one drug in the majority of hypertensive patients has also become obvious. This is nowhere better seen than among elderly diabetic hypertensive patients, who will be considered in the next section. Therefore, the best combination of agents, almost always to include a low dose of diuretic, will be a more pertinent object of trials in the future.

Drugs for specific indications

A variety of comorbid conditions that are often seen in elderly hypertensives may be favorably influenced by one class of drug or another, whereas others may be adversely affected by certain drugs. These individualized choices are based on clinical experience, but most do not have the support of RCTs that would make their use 'compelling'. However, the wisdom of using an α-blocker to relieve the symptoms of prostatism while also lowering the blood pressure is obvious. As noted by Lieber (1998), α-blockade is now the accepted initial therapy for most patients with urinary obstructive symptoms, so that only one drug will often manage the two conditions, hypertension and BPH, which occur together in as many as 25 of elderly men. Concerns about α-blockers arising from the termination of that arm of the ALLHAT trial because of an apparent increased incidence of heart failure compared to the diuretic arm (ALLHAT, 2000) should not deny their use along with a low dose of diuretic when indicated.

ACEIs and ARBs are clearly indicated for diabetic hypertensive patients (Hostetter, 2001). If one of these agents is not sufficient to bring the blood pressure to below 130/80 mmHg, a low dose of thiazide is the next logical step. If the blood pressure is still too high, a calcium antagonist may be required.

Patients with renal insufficiency, defined as a serum creatinine above 1.5 mg/dl, almost always need a larger dose of more potent loop diuretics to overcome the sodium retention that is largely responsible for the progressive hypertension seen with worsening renal function. ACEIs are always indicated. If diabetic nephropathy is the cause of renal damage, an ARB may be chosen instead. Most will require a third drug, and a calcium antagonist is often the best choice to control hypertension.

Special guidelines for the elderly

These recommendations should be helpful in controlling hypertension in the elderly, in addition to those described later that are aimed at improving overall compliance with therapy (Kaplan, 2002).

1. Always check for postural and postprandial hypotension before starting antihypertensive drug therapy to avoid even more precipitous falls in blood pressure. If present, utilize the various maneuvers described earlier to overcome the postural and postprandial falls in blood pressure.

2. Establish the goal of therapy as 140/85 mmHg or lower; those with coronary disease should not have their diastolics reduced below 80 mmHg; those with ISH should have their systolics reduced to 140 mmHg, but with concern about lowering of diastolic blood pressure to below 65 mmHg; those with diabetes or renal insufficiency should have their blood pressure reduced below 130/80 mmHg.

3. Start with a low dose of a thiazide diuretic, preferably in combination with a potassium-sparing agent; if the serum creatinine is above 1.5 mg/dl, metolazone once daily or multiple daily doses of furosemide or torsemide may be needed.

4. If the diuretic is inadequate or poorly tolerated, add or substitute a long-acting DHP calcium antagonist, again starting with a dose one-half the usual starting dose. Titrate slowly, every 4–8 weeks, until control is attained.

5. Use agents in addition to diuretics or DHP calcium antagonists that provide favorable influences on comorbid conditions, as noted in Figure 34.

6. If a β-blocker is indicated, as with angina or post myocardial infarction, or an alpha-blocker for prostatism, always add a low dose of thiazide diuretic.

7. Always use once-a-day dosing with long-acting agents that provide full 24-hour efficacy. Agents such as amlodipine and trandolapril, with inherently longer durations of action, are particularly attractive to cover the days when doses are skipped – a common occurrence.

8. Home monitoring of the blood pressure is extremely useful both to ensure adequate 24-hour control by having early morning readings prior to the day's therapy and to avoid the office white-coat effect, which may lead to inadvertent overtreatment. Office readings that are high because of the white-coat effect may cause the patient's hypertension to appear to be under-treated when it is in fact well controlled or even overtreated.

9. Avoid drug interactions that are more common in the elderly, as they often take a number of different types of medication (Rochon and Gurwitz, 1997). Some, such as grapefruit juice, potentiate antihypertensive effects, but the most common interaction is with non-steroidal anti-inflammatory agents (NSAIDs), which will antagonize the effects of all agents save calcium antagonists (Harris and Brater, 2001). As noted by Johnson (1998), about 15% of elderly hypertensives take an NSAID and antihypertensive drugs concurrently. Johnson recommends the use of physical therapy and other analgesics such as aceta-minophen, which do not interfere with anti-hypertensive drug efficacy.

Erectile dysfunction

Erectile dysfunction is common in elderly men, usually a consequence of atherosclerotic impairment of penile blood flow. Hypertension may add to the problem, which may be further aggravated by antihypertensive therapy. As reported by Grimm et al. (1997), of the five classes of antihypertensives compared in the Treatment of Mild Hypertension Study (TOMHS), only diuretics significantly increased the incidence of erectile impotence. Only 15 mg of chlorthalidone was used, so the problem can obviously be exacerbated by low doses of diuretics.

Until sildenafil (Viagra) became available, erectile dysfunction that began after antihypertensive therapy was begun was usually best managed by stopping the drug(s) being given, waiting for the return of potency and restarting therapy with a low dose of another class of drug. Now the best course, if the antihypertensive therapy is otherwise effective and well tolerated, may be to simply give sildenafil, which should have no interaction with any antihypertensive drug. Caution is obviously needed to avoid the use of sildenafil with nitrates that may induce profound hypotension.

Even if all the guidelines are followed, compliance with therapy may be poor. Advice to improve compliance is provided next.

Improving compliance

Fewer than half of patients begun on antihypertensive therapy will still be taking their medication after 1 year. According to a survey of over 1000 hypertensives in England reported by Jones et al. (1995), the continuation rates at 6 months were between 40 and 50% regardless of the class of antihypertensive drug prescribed. On the other hand, Monane et al. (1997) found better compliance with other classes than with diuretics among a group of 8600 elderly hypertensives enrolled in the New Jersey Medicare program from 1982 to 1988. Compliance worsened when multiple drugs were prescribed and improved with more physician visits.

Unfortunately, hypertension and its treatment fulfill many of the criteria that are known to reduce adherence to any therapy (Table 17). As hypertension is an asymptomatic,

Patient and disease characteristics
Asymptomatic
Chronic condition
Condition suppressed, not cured
No immediate consequences of stopping therapy
Social isolation
Disrupted home situation
Psychiatric illness

Treatment characteristics
Long duration of therapy
Complicated regimens
Expensive medications
Side effects of medications
Multiple behavioral modifications
Lack of specific appointment times
Long waiting time in office

Table 17 Factors that reduce adherence to therapy

Be aware of the problem and be alert to signs of patient non-adherence

Establish the goal of therapy: to reduce blood pressure to near normotensive levels with minimal or no side effects

Educate the patient about the disease and its treatment
Involve the patient in decision making
Encourage family support

Maintain contact with the patient
Encourage visits and calls to allied health personnel
Allow the pharmacist to monitor therapy
Give feedback to the patient via home BP readings
Make contact with patients who do not return

Keep care inexpensive and simple
Do the least workup needed to rule out secondary causes
Obtain follow-up laboratory data only yearly unless indicated more often
Use home blood pressure readings
Use non-drug, low-cost therapies
Use once-daily doses of long-acting drugs
Use generic drugs and break larger doses of tables in half
If appropriate, use combination tablets
Tailor medication to daily routines

Prescribe according to pharmacological principles
Add one drug at a time
Start with small doses, aiming for 5–10 mmHg reductions at each step
Have medication taken immediately on awakening in the morning or after 4 am if patient wakes to void
Prevent volume overload with adequate diuretic and sodium restriction

Be willing to stop unsuccessful therapy and try a different approach

Anticipate side effects

Adjust therapy to ameliorate side effects that do not disappear spontaneously

Continue to add effective and tolerated drugs, stepwise, in sufficient doses to achieve the goal of therapy

Table 18 General guidelines to improve patient adherence to antihypertensive therapy

chronic incurable condition whose treatment requires daily therapy that may cause side effects and which provides no obvious benefit, it is easy to see why so few patients adhere closely to their therapy.

Table 18 provides general guidelines to improve patient compliance with therapy. Unfortunately, few of these have been documented to be successful. In their review of all published randomized trials of interventions to improve compliance Haynes et al. (1996) could identify only 13 that met their criteria for an adequate study design. Five of these involved hypertensives. Improved adherence to antihypertensive therapy was noted with these interventions.

- One dose of drug/day compared to two doses/day
- Tailoring of therapy to individual patients
- Self-monitoring of pills and blood pressure
- Rewards for higher adherence and lower blood pressure
- Worksite care by nurses

These findings support the use of home blood pressure readings, simplified once-daily regimens that fit the individual patient's needs, and easy access to convenient care. The elderly often have additional impediments to adherence to therapy, ranging from difficulty in opening childproof containers to an inability to pay for expensive drugs, to difficulty in reaching their healthcare providers.

Hopefully, the guidelines provided in Table 18 and elsewhere in this book will help physicians and their patients to achieve the true goal of antihypertensive therapy: to control hypertension without adverse effects that interfere with the quality of life while providing protection from hypertension-induced cardiovascular morbidity and mortality.

References

Alderman MH, Cohen H, Madhavan S. Dietary sodium intake and mortality: the National Health and Nutrition Examination Survey (NHANES I). *Lancet* 1998;**351**:781–5.

ALLHAT Officers and Coordinators for the ALLHAT Collaborative Research Group. Major cardiovascular events in hypertensive patients randomized to doxazosin vs chlorthalidone. The Antihypertensive and Lipid-Lowering Treatment to Prevent Heart Attack Trial (ALLHAT). *JAMA* 2000;**283**:1967–75.

Appel LJ, Espeland MA, Easter L, Wilson AC, Folmar S, Lacy CR. Effects of reduced sodium intake on hypertension control in older individuals. *Arch Intern Med* 2001;**161**:685–93.

Barker DJP. Fetal origins of coronary heart disease. *Br Med J* 1995;**311**:171–4.

Beevers G, Lip GYH, O'Brien E. Blood pressure measurement. Part I – Sphygmomanometry: Factors common to all techniques. *Br Med J* 2001;**322**:981–5.

Blood Pressure Lowering Treatment Trialists' Collaboration. Effects of ACE inhibitors, calcium antagonists, and other blood-pressure-lowering drugs: results of prospectively designed overviews of randomised trials. *Lancet* 2000;**356**:1955–64.

Brenner BM, Chertow GM. Congenital oligonephropathy and the etiology of adult hypertension and progressive renal injury. *Am J Kidney Dis* 1994;**23**:171–5.

British Hypertension Society. Technique of blood pressure measurement. *Hypertension* 1985;**3**:293.

Brown MJ, Palmer CR, Castaigne A et al. Morbidity and mortality in patients randomised to double-blind treatment with a long-acting calcium-channel blocker or diuretic in the International Nifedipine GITS study: Intervention as a Goal in Hypertension Treatment (INSIGHT). *Lancet* 2000;**356**:366–72.

Buck C, Baker P, Bass M, Donner A. The prognosis of hypertension according to age at onset. *Hypertension* 1987;**9**:204–8.

Burt VL, Whelton P, Roccella EJ et al. Prevalence of hypertension in the US adult population. Results from the Third National Health and Nutrition Examination Survey 1988–91. *Hypertension* 1995;**25**:305–13.

Cutler JA, Follman D, Allender PS. Randomized trials of sodium reduction: an overview. *Am J Clin Nutr* 1997;**65**(Suppl):643S–51S.

Dodson PM, Lip GYH, Eames SM et al. Hypertensive retinopathy: a review of existing classification systems and a suggestion for a simplified grading system. *J Hum Hypertens* 1996;**10**:93–98.

Epstein FH. Primary prevention of coronary heart disease. *Excerpta Med* 1980;**I**:1–11.

Estacio RO, Jeffers BW, Hiatt WR et al. The effect of nisoldipine as compared with enalapril on cardiovascular outcomes in patients with non-insulin-dependent diabetes and hypertension. *N Engl J Med* 1998;**338**:645–52.

Forette F, Seux M-L, Staessen JA et al. Prevention of dementia in randomised double-blind placebo-controlled systolic hypertension in Europe (Syst-Eur) trial. *Lancet* 1998;**352**:1347–51.

Franklin SS, Larson MG, Khan SA et al. Does the relation of blood pressure to coronary heart disease risk change with aging? The Framingham Heart Study. *Circulation* 2001a;**103**:1245–9.

Franklin SS, Jacobs MJ, Wong ND, L'Italien GJ, Lapuerta P. Predominance of isolated systolic hypertension among middle-aged and elderly US hypertensives: analysis based on national health and nutrition examination survey (NHANES) III. *Hypertension* 2001b;**37**:869–74.

Gong L, Zhang W, Zhy Y et al. Shanghai trial of nifedipine in the elderly (STONE). *J Hypertens* 1996;**14**:1237–45.

Goode GK, Miller JP, Heagerty AM. Hyperlipidaemia, hypertension, and coronary heart disease. *Lancet* 1995;**345**:362–4.

Grimm RH, Grandits GA, Prineas RJ et al. Long-term effects on sexual function of five antihypertensive drugs and nutritional hygienic treatment in hypertensive men and women. *Hypertension* 1997;**29**:8–14.

Grodzicki T, Rajzer M, Fagard R et al. Ambulatory blood pressure monitoring and postprandial hypotension in elderly patients with isolated systolic hypertension. *J Hum Hypertens* 1998;**12**:161–5.

Groppelli A, Giorgi DMA, Omboni S, Parati G, Mancia G. Persistent blood pressure increase induced by heavy smoking. *J Hypertens* 1992;**10**:495–9.

Grossman E, Messerli FH. Effect of calcium antagonists on plasma norepinephrine levels, heart rate, and blood pressure. *Am J Cardiol* 1997;**80**:1453–8.

Gueyffier F, Bulpitt C, Boissel J-P et al. Antihypertensive drugs in very old people: a subgroup meta-analysis of randomised controlled trials. *Lancet* 1999;**353**:793–6.

Guidelines Subcommittee. 1999 World Health Organization [WHO] - International Society of Hypertension guidelines for the management of hypertension. *J Hypertens* 1999;**17**:151–83.

Hakim AA, Petrovitch H, Burchfiel CM et al. Effects of walking on mortality among nonsmoking retired men. *N Engl J Med* 1998;**338**:94–9.

Hall CL, Higgs CMB, Notarianni L. Home blood pressure recording in mild hypertension: value of distinguishing sustained from clinic hypertension and effect on diagnosis and treatment. *J Hum Hypertens* 1990;**4**:501–7.

Hallock P, Benson IC. Studies of the elastic properties of human isolated aorta. *J Clin Invest* 1937;**16**:595–602.

Hansson L, Zanchetti A, Carruthers SG et al. Benefits of intensive blood pressure lowering and acetylsalicylic acid in hypertensive patients. Principal results of the Hypertension Optimal Treatment (HOT) Study. *Lancet* 1998;**351**:1755–62.

Hansson L, Lindholm LH, Ekbom T et al. Randomized trial of old and new antihypertensive drugs in elderly patients: cardiovascular mortality and morbidity in the Swedish Trial in Old Patients with Hypertension-2 study. *Lancet* 1999;**354**:1751–6.

Harris CJ, Brater DC. Renal effects of cyclooxygenase-2 selective inhibitors. *Curr Opin Nephrol Hypertens* 2001;**10**:603–10.

Haynes RB, McKibbon KA, Kanani R. Systematic review of randomised trials of interventions to assist patients to follow prescriptions for medications. *Lancet* 1996;**348**:383–6.

He FJ, Whelton PK. Selection of initial antihypertensive drug therapy. *Lancet* 2000;**356**:1942–3.

He FJ, MacGregor GA. Beneficial effects of potassium. *Br Med J* 2001;**323**:497–501.

Heart Outcomes Prevention Evaluation (HOPE) Study Investigators. Effects of an angiotensin-converting-enzyme inhibitor, ramipril, on death from cardiovascular causes, myocardial infarction, and stroke in high-risk patients. *N Engl J Med* 2000;**342**:145–53.

Hostetter TH. Prevention of end-stage renal disease due to type 2 diabetes. *N Engl J Med* 2001;**345**:910–12.

Huang Z, Willett WC, Manson JE. Body weight, weight change and risk for hypertension in women. *Ann Intern Med* 1998;**128**:81–8.

Jackson R, Barham P, Biels J et al. Management of raised blood pressure in New Zealand: a discussion document. *Br Med J* 1993;**307**:107–10.

Johnson AG. NSAIDS and blood pressure. *Drugs Aging* 1998;**12**:17–27.

Joint National Committee. The sixth report of the Joint National Committee on Detection, Evaluation, and Treatment of High Blood Pressure (JNC-VI). *Arch Intern Med* 1997;**157**:2413–46.

Jones JK, Gorkin L, Lian JF et al. Discontinuation of and changes in treatment after start of new courses of antihypertensive drugs: a study of a United Kingdom population. *Br Med J* 1995;**311**:293–5.

Joshipura KJ, Ascherio A, Manson JE et al. Fruit and vegetable intake in relation to risk of ischemic stroke. *JAMA* 1999;**282**:1233–9.

Kannel WB. Prospects for prevention of cardiovascular disease in the elderly. *Prev Cardiol* 1998;**1**:32–9.

Kannel WB. Elevated systolic blood pressure as a cardiovascular risk factor. *Am J Cardiol* 2000;**85**:251–5.

Kaplan NM. Primary Hypertension: Pathogenesis. In: Kaplan NM, ed. *Clinical hypertension*, 8th edn. Philadelphia: Lippincott Williams & Wilkins, 2002.

Keith NM, Wagener HP, Barker NW. Some different types of essential hypertension: their course and prognosis. *Am J Med Sci* 1937;**197**:332–43.

Kizer JR, Kimmel SE. Epidemiologic review of the calcium channel blocker drugs. An up-to-date perspective on the proposed hazards. *Arch Intern Med* 2001;**161**:1145–58.

Lavie P, Hoffstein V. Sleep apnea syndrome: a possible contributing factor to resistant hypertension. *SLEEP* 2001;**24**:721.

Lieber MM. Pharmacologic therapy for prostatism. *Mayo Clin Proc* 1998;**73**:590–6.

Lipsitz LA, Stouch HA, Manikear KL, Rowe JW. Intra-individual variability in postural BP in the elderly. *Clin Sci* 1985;**69**:337–41.

Liu L, Wang JG, Gong L et al., for the Systolic Hypertension in China (Syst-China) Collaborative Group. Comparison of active treatment and placebo in older Chinese patients with isolated systolic hypertension. *J Hypertens* 1998;**16**:1823–9.

MacMahon S, Peto R, Cutler J et al. Blood pressure, stroke, and coronar heart disease, Part 1: Prolonged differences in blood pressure. *Lance* 1990;**335**:765–74.

Mancia G, Sega R, Milesi C et al. Blood pressure control in the hyper tensive population. *Lancet* 1997;**349**:454–7.

Messerli FH, Grossman E, Goldburt U. Are β-blockers efficacious as first line therapy for hypertension in the elderly? *JAMA* 1998;**279**:1903–7

Monane M, Bohn RL, Gurwitz JH et al. The effects of initial drug choic and comorbidity on antihypertensive therapy compliance. *Am J Hyper tens* 1997;**10**:697–704.

Morgan TO, Anderson AIE, MacInnis RJ. ACE inhibitors, beta-blockers calcium blockers, and diuretics for the control of systolic hypertensior *Am J Hypertens* 2001;**14**:241–7.

Neaton JD, Wentworth D. Serum cholesterol blood pressure, cigarett smoking and death from coronary heart disease. Overall findings an differences by age for 316,099 white men. *Arch Intern Me* 1992;**152**:56–64.

O'Brien E. Ave atque vale: the centenary of clinical sphygmomanometry *Lancet* 1996;**348**:1569–70.

Ofili EO, Cohen JD, St. Vrain JA et al. Effect of treatment of isolate systolic hypertension on left ventricular mass. *JAMA* 1998;**279**:778–8C

O'Rourke M. Mechanical principles in arterial disease. *Hypertensio* 1995;**26**:2–9.

Pickering TG. Blood pressure monitoring outside the office for th evaluation of patients with resistant hypertension. *Hypertensio* 1988;**11**(Suppl II):II96–II100.

PROGRESS Collaborative Group. Randomised trial of a perindopril-base blood-pressure-lowering regimen among 6105 individuals with previ ous stroke or transient ischaemic attack. *Lancet* 2001;**358**:1033–41.

Psaty BM, Smith NL, Siscovick DS et al. Health outcomes associated witl antihypertensive therapies used as first-line agents. *JAM* 1997;**277**:739–45.

Ramsay LE, Williams B, Johnston GD et al. British Hypertension Societ guidelines for hypertension management 1999: summary. *Br Med* 1999;**319**:630–5.

Rochon PA, Gurwitz JH. Optimizing drug treatment for elderly people the prescribing cascade. *Br Med J* 1997;**315**:1096–9.

Sacks FM, Willett WC, Smith A et al. Effect on blood pressure of potas sium, calcium and magnesium in women with low habitual intake *Hypertension* 1998;**31**:131–8.

Sacks FM, Svetkey LP, Vollmer WM et al. Effects on blood pressure o reduced dietary sodium and the Dietary Approaches to Stop Hyper tension (DASH) diet. *N Engl J Med* 2001;**344**:3–10.

Satish S, Freeman DH, Ray L, Goodwin JS. The relationship between bloo pressure and mortality in the oldest old. *J Am Geriatr So* 2001;**49**:367–74.

Savage PJ, Pressel SL, Curb JD et al. Influence of long-term, low-dose diuretic-based, antihypertension therapy on glucose, lipid, uric acid and potassium levels in older men and women with isolated systoli hypertension. *Arch Intern Med* 1998;**158**:741–51.

Schwartz SM, Ross R. Cellular proliferation in atherosclerosis and hyper tension. *Prog Cardiovasc Dis* 1985;**26**:355.

haper AG, Wannamethee G, Whincup P. Alcohol and blood pressure in middle aged British men. *J Hum Hypertens* 1988;**2**:71–8.

HEP Cooperative Research Group. Prevention of stroke by antihypertensive drug treatment in older persons with isolated systolic hypertension. *JAMA* 1991;**265**:3255–64.

omes GW, Pahor M, Shorr RI et al. The role of diastolic blood pressure when treating isolated systolic hypertension. *Arch Intern Med* 1999;**159**:2004–9.

aessen JA, Fagard R, Lijnen P, Amery A. Body weight, sodium intake and blood pressure. *J Hypertens* 1989;**7**(Suppl 1):19–23.

aessen JA, Fagard R, Thijs L et al. Randomized double-blind comparison of placebo and active treatment of older patients with isolated systolic hypertension. *Lancet* 1997;**350**:757–64.

aessen JA, Gasowski J, Wang JG et al. Risks of untreated and treated isolated systolic hypertension in the elderly: meta-analysis of outcome trials. *Lancet* 2000;**355**:865–72.

aessen JA, Wang J-G, Thijs L. Cardiovascular protection and blood pressure reduction. *Lancet* 2001;**358**:1305–15.

tewart IMG. Relation of reduction in pressure to first myocardial infarction in patients receiving treatment for severe hypertension. *Lancet* 1979;**1**:1861–5.

hun MJ, Peto R, Lopez AD et al. Alcohol consumption and mortality among middle-aged and elderly U.S. adults. *N Engl J Med* 1997;**337**:1705–14.

onkin AL. Postural hypotension. *Med J Aust* 1995;**162**:436–8.

an Jaarsveld BC, Krijnen P, Pieterman H et al., for the Dutch Renal Artery Stenosis Intervention Cooperative Study Group. The effects of balloon angioplasty on hypertension in atherosclerotic renal-artery stenosis. *N Engl J Med* 2000;**342**:1007–14.

asbinder GBC, Nelemans PJ, Kessels AGH et al. Diagnostic tests for renal artery stenosis in patients suspected of having renovascular hypertension: a meta-analysis. *Ann Intern Med* 2001;**135**:401–11.

erdecchia P. Using out of office blood pressure monitoring in the management of hypertension. *Curr Hypertension Rep* 2001;**3**:400–5.

erdecchia P, Schillaci G, Boldrini F et al. White coat hypertension. *Lancet* 1996;**348**:1443–5.

okó Z, Bots ML, Hofman A et al. J-shaped relation between blood pressure and stroke in treated hypertensives. *Hypertension* 1999;**34**:1181–5.

einberger MH, Fineberg NS. Sodium and volume sensitivity of blood pressure. Age and pressure change over time. *Hypertension* 1991;**18**:67–71.

einberger MH, Fineberg NS, Fineberg SE, Weinberger M. Salt sensitivity, pulse pressure, and death in normal and hypertensive humans. Hypertension 2001;**37**:429–32.

Vhelton PK, Appel LJ, Espeland MA et al. Sodium reduction and weight loss in the treatment of hypertension in older persons. *JAMA* 1998;**279**:839–46.

achariah PK, Sheps SG, Smith RL. Defining the roles of home and ambulatory monitoring. *Diagnosis* 1988;**10**:39–50.

Index